# How To Win Clients
# And Interpret Their Needs

# How To Win Clients
## And Interpret Their Needs

A Hairdresser's Guide

## Ian Mistlin

OXFORD

BLACKWELL SCIENTIFIC PUBLICATIONS

LONDON EDINBURGH BOSTON

MELBOURNE PARIS BERLIN VIENNA

© Ian Mistlin 1994

Blackwell Scientific Publications
Editorial Offices:
Osney Mead, Oxford OX2 0EL
25 John Street, London WC1N 2BL
23 Ainslie Place, Edinburgh EH3 6AJ
238 Main Street, Cambridge,
  Massachusetts 02142, USA
54 University Street, Carlton,
  Victoria 3053, Australia

  Other Editorial Offices:
  Librairie Arnette SA
  1, rue de Lille
  75007 Paris
  France

  Blackwell Wissenschafts-Verlag GmbH
  Kurfürskendamm 57
  10707 Berlin
  Germany

  Blackwell MZV
  Feldgasse 13
  A-1238 Wien
  Austria

First published 1994

Set by DP Photosetting, Aylesbury, Bucks
Printed and bound in Great Britain by
Hartnolls Ltd, Bodmin, Cornwall

DISTRIBUTORS

Marston Book Services Ltd
PO Box 87
Oxford OX2 0DT
(*Orders:* Tel: 0865 791155
        Fax: 0865 791927
        Telex: 837515)

USA
  Blackwell Scientific Publications, Inc.
  238 Main Street
  Cambridge, MA 02142
  (*Orders:* Tel: 800 759-6102
          617 876-7000)

Canada
  Oxford University Press
  70 Wynford Drive
  Don Mills
  Ontario M3C 1J9
  (*Orders:* Tel: (416) 441-2941)

Australia
  Blackwell Scientific Publications Pty Ltd
  54 University Street
  Carlton, Victoria 3053
  (*Orders:* Tel: 03 347-5552)

British Library
Cataloguing in Publication Data
A Catalogue record for this book is available from
the British Library

ISBN 0–632–03891–8

Library of Congress
Cataloging in Publication Data
Mistlin, Ian.
    How to win clients and interpret their needs:
a hairdresser's guide/Ian Mistlin.
      p.  cm.
    Includes index.
    ISBN 0-632-03891-8
    1. Beauty shops—Management.   2. Beauty
shops—Marketing.   3. Beauty shops—
Customer services.   I. Title.
TT965.M57   1994
646.7′2′068—dc20                    94-17887
                                    CIP

# Contents

# Acknowledgements

To my wife, Glenda, parents and family for their constant support.

To my sons, Jamie and Dean, may you always be winners.

To Paul Aldous for his design talents.

To Sue Butt for her secretarial services.

To Richard Miles of Blackwell Scientific Publications for his publisher's confidence.

To my former work colleagues, now worldwide, a big hello!

# *Introduction*

What plans do you make each year? Do you plan ahead? What is your sales potential? Do you regularly take stock of your career direction? I'm sure you have set yourself objectives in the hope that it will bring you new challenges, success, job satisfaction and self-fulfilment.

At a time when the country is gripped with recession and we see business closures, a slump in sales and the coming down of European trade barriers, the success of many businesses will depend on how quickly they can adjust to the social, political and economic changes.

Hairdressing is no exception. The fittest individuals and salons will survive. Survival will demand constant attention and responsiveness to your clients' needs. Success in the 1990s and beyond will be determined by your willingness to change and by your being adequately prepared to meet these needs, through a programme of continuous improvement.

Personal growth and self-improvement in hairdressing will only be achieved through continuous learning. Experience counts: you must build upon a solid foundation of core skills and have dedication and a determination to achieve new goals.

Salon growth will reflect a growing trend towards developing and nurturing a quality culture.

Recognizing the importance of these issues, *How to Win Clients and Interpret Their Needs* explores the complex subject of how to *sense, sell, serve* and *satisfy* the needs and expectations of your clients. The book is about looking, listening, communicating and interpreting your clients' needs.

Hairdressing is an adventure, a journey rich in rewards, but unless care is taken there can be many pitfalls and hurdles en route. Success depends on what route you take.

My goal is to take the subject matter on to the shop floor and share with you my experience and expertise. The book provides essential reading material for all college students, salon trainees, and newly qualified and established hairdressers, who, although at different stages in their careers, are looking to:

- successfully market their services;
- appreciate the art of selling;
- increase sales potential;
- improve client relationships;
- create a positive business image;
- make those first impressions count;
- enhance personal presentation;
- practise effective communication;
- discover the secrets of body language;
- improve vocal image;
- polish consultation techniques;
- build a quality service.

It will also be of value to lecturers, managers and salon owners who are in a position to bring about change.

To the trainee: you are the stars of tomorrow.

To the newly qualified hairdresser: some day you may plan to open your own salon, but first you need to know the basics.

To the qualified hairdresser: one is never too old to learn or make changes and open new doors.

To the lecturer: you are educating the stars of tomorrow.

To the salon manager: your team will be looking to you for those touches of creative management.

To the salon owner: you are the 'captain of the ship', responsible for managing rewards.

I cannot offer you any short cuts, but what I can offer are a number of routes to make your journey less hazardous and more rewarding.

# PART I
# DEVELOP YOUR CLIENT MARKETING

# 1
# A Marketing Overview

I take up the journey some years back when I was at a business seminar on marketing. I recall the very words the speaker used.

> A business can have good products, adequate financing, competent managers, an excellent location, comfortable interiors, effective advertising and PR . . . and still fail.

After this he paused for a few moments and then continued,

> A business cannot be successful without happy and satisfied customers. They are your greatest asset. Without them it would be impossible to earn your livelihood. Clients are the boss.

These are wise words. A salon without clients would not be in business for long. It's the clients who are paying the wages. As one customer remarked to an unhelpful sales assistant, 'I believe you have things backwards. You are overhead, I am profit.' This can be applied to any business that relies on customers, and is central to good marketing.

**Marketing** is about products and markets. A **product** is something that a company sells: a conventional product, such as a car; a service, for example car maintenance; or something in between, such as hair design produced by a salon for its customers, where the salon is also providing a service. **Markets** are customer groupings which could theoretically be supplied by the company. If the company is selling cars, it could in theory supply all the cars purchased in the town or country, in Europe or in the world. In reality it would be wiser for that company to concentrate on an accessible market. This is the market that the company can logistically serve, taking into consideration its marketing strength; the demand; its output; whether it can produce sufficient quantities to meet the demand;

the ability of the workforce to cope; the availability of sufficient financial and technological resources; whether the market will bear the price; and how the product will be distributed. The larger the company gets, the more complex becomes it marketing concept.

Marketing is a concept and a series of activities concerned with

- the product or service
- promotion
- pricing
- distribution (or place).

Other activities that can be included are

- market research
- market planning
- packaging
- personal selling.

All these activities form part of what we call the **marketing mix** which can be split into:

**Front-line marketing activities**, which are seen as visible outputs to the customer. These include:

- product development
- promotion
- pricing
- selling
- service.

**Behind-the-line marketing**, which mostly goes on behind the scenes. These inputs are:

- market, customer and product research
- planning.

Each company must decide on the right mix to suit its needs, and incorporate them together with its marketing concept into the marketing plan. It is all very well having a plan, but behind the best plans of battle there must be a strategy for attacking, consolidating or defending one's current position. Military precision is needed, and you must have a clear, well thought out marketing strategy to shape the plan.

# Who needs a marketing strategy?

The answer is every company, business, organization or individual which has a mission and a will to survive and generate controlled, profitable, long-term growth. Such growth can only be achieved if the customers' needs are identified, anticipated and met.

# What are the rewards?

Success can be measured by:

- satisfied customers;
- referrals from existing customers;
- prospective customers;
- a return on investment;
- increased turnover (although this does not always mean increased profits, which can be greatly affected by overheads).

## Out with the old

In the traditional concept of marketing, the product manufacturer who wanted to increase sales would simply develop a new product and then sell it in the same way, in the same outlets as other products. The customer in this scenario would be on the outside and the company would be inward looking.

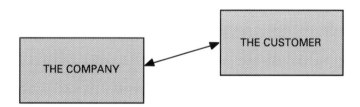

## In with the new

Many companies have now replaced this by a customer-centred approach which puts the customer at the very centre of the organization.

Here a company would not rely solely on its own judgement about what product to develop but would ask the customers what they wanted. Their ideas and suggestions are sought by first using market research techniques, so that new products can be tailored to consumers' needs.

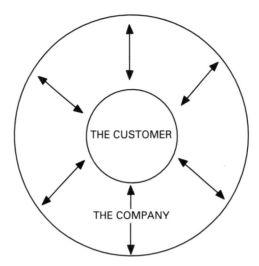

Customer satisfaction is then measured by communicating directly with the customer. Developing this circular relationship between the producer and the customer gives a producer more confidence and a greater chance of success in the market-place.

**Client-centred marketing** is a technique that you can use to advance your traditional marketing approach and develop a unique relationship with:

- your existing clientele
- referral sources
- targets of opportunity.

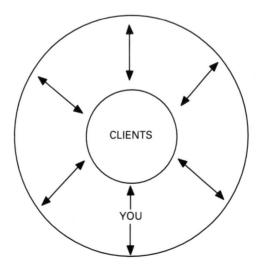

## Bank the benefits

Look upon this marketing approach as a form of investment that will produce a profitable return on your initial outlay, your time, and your human and financial resources.

You may argue that this approach is going to take up more of your time. On the contrary: utilizing your time more effectively and efficiently enables you to produce the greatest number of results and rewards from the smallest number of actions. These include:

- exploiting your existing client potential;
- increasing your target opportunities;
- attacking your competition;
- improved sales.

I will now provide an outline on how to get started on the decisive elements of your strategic marketing.

# The elements of client-centred marketing

*Define the mission of your salon.* This is a statement that consists of answers to the questions:

- What do you do?
- What do you provide?
- Whom do you provide to?
- How do you provide?

*Define your salon's purpose, i.e. objectives.* This requires a statement that defines your salon's service commitment to your clients. It needs to state clearly what your salon specifically intends to provide to your clients, and the values that exist within your salon.

*Plan your attack.* Analyse your market opportunities, in order to sense whether the relationship is going to be fruitful. This is done by:

- analysing and segmenting your client sources, so that their requirements can be identified;
- identifying who your competitors might be and their strengths and weaknesses;
- focusing on environmental trends that may affect your market;
- conducting an inventory of your salon's strengths and weaknesses so that you stand a chance of meeting market requirements;

- instigating market research to test your market opportunities;
- deciding on what promotion methods to use to reach the market.

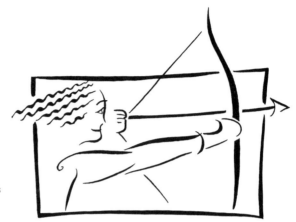

Plan your attack: is
your attack well
aimed?

## Client sources

Your client sources are made up of the following.

### Your existing clientele

Your regular clients offer an opportunity for potential growth. They may have unmet needs and may be interested in additional services you offer.

### Referral sources

- Regular clients who are happy with your services can provide you with valuable new leads, as well as written testimonials.
- Business contacts who are not clients but nevertheless know of your reputation can be used to supply you with new leads.

### Targets of opportunity or prospects

This category includes:

- Latent, effective or potential client types who have been identified and could theoretically be interested in your services.
- Any prospective client whom you have met recently during a talk or demonstration or following a walk-in consultation.
- Previously regular clients whom you have not seen for some time.

■ Those groups of clients who receive discounts for whatever reason. They need to be monitored.

## *Prospecting*

This process is concerned with identifying those individuals, markets or niches which could theoretically be interested in your services. Not all clients will have the same need for your services, so they must be analysed and segmented so that specific needs for each can be identified and understood. Knowing what your market opportunities are, who are likely to want your services, is not something you can do by pure guesswork. It requires market research to separate those segments into distinguishable segments and characteristics that:

■ are accessible to your marketing strategy;
■ can sustain business growth;
■ can separate you from your competitors.

The segments may be described by:

■ the type of demand;
■ the differences in the benefits sought;
■ the availability of alternative means of satisfying their needs through choice.

## Demand

Throughout this marketing overview I will constantly refer to **demand**. What is it? Demand is a term used by economists to describe consumer behaviour. It can be separated into the following categories:

▢ **Effective demand:** This is used to express a demand for a service or product backed up by purchasing power.

▢ **Latent demand:** This can be defined as a demand for a service or product which clients are unable to satisfy, usually for lack of purchasing power. For example, many clients may have a want for a colouring service but in view of their available disposable income it may not be high on their list of priorities. Latent demand can also arise out of a client's want for a particular service or product which is unavailable.

▢ **Potential demand:** This exists where a client possesses the necessary purchasing power but is not currently buying services.

The overall aim is to use your marketing strategy to move the client through the following stages:

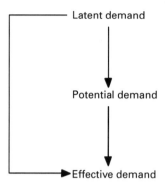

Latent demand

Potential demand

Effective demand

This is done by:

- promotional activities;
- reducing prices (not to be recommended);
- increasing clients' perception of value (a must).

## Competition

I have already discussed demand as a measure of customer behaviour. On the other side of the equation is **supply**. This describes the nature of the market, that is, how many sellers there are supplying the same or similar services. These sellers pose a threat to your existence. They are your competition, for in theory they offer choice.

**Choice** means a single benefit or set of benefits that may attract clients to seek them out.

- Do you know the competition in your trading location?
- Do you know what services they are offering?
- Do you know your competitors' strengths and weaknesses?
- Do you know how much they are charging?
- Do you know what client type seeks them out?
- Do you know how many staff they have?
- Do you know their hours and days of trading?
- Do you know how they attract business?

If you do not have the answers to these important questions, you need to find them out.

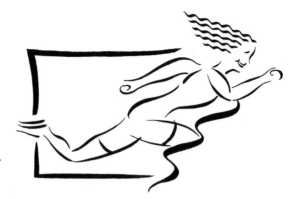

Competition: going for
gold.

## Who are your clients?

To answer this accurately you will need to consider what determines a
demand and how you can build up a profile of your clients by analysing
them into segments or characteristics based on socio-economic and
psychological environmental trends. This method of segmentation can be
summarized as follows.

### *Geographic segments*

Clients are your basic raw material, so it is essential to know where they
come from.

- Do you have an international clientele?
- Is your salon located in a city, a county town or a rural community?
- If you draw from any of these places or surrounding areas, what is the
  density of their populations?
- If your clients travel to you from far afield, what are the transport
  facilities like?
- How far will they be prepared to travel?
- Will climatic conditions deter clients from booking?
- If you rely on walk-in trade, are you well positioned?

### *Demographic segments*

What effect will age, sex, family size and income have on your market? It
will be important to consider these questions:

- Which age group has the potential for greatest growth?
- What is the size of this age group within your reach?

- What is the size of this age group nationally?
- Where are they concentrated?
- What about other age groups?
- Can these groups be broken down into male and female?
- From number profiles, which sex is more dominant?
- How will these figures compare in the future?
- Do you know the ratio of single to married people?
- In a family unit how many incomes are there?
- How much disposable income is there?
- What about educational background?
- Are they employed (if so, what is their occupation?), unemployed or retired?
- Are they planning to return to work?
- Do they have small children?
- How do these figures pan out locally and nationally?

## Socio-cultural characteristics

If your business is international, are you aware of cultural needs based on beliefs, values, attitudes and habits?

Are you aware of any subcultures within your business community? If so, what issues will be of importance? Will they be based on race, religion or nationality?

Although you may not wish to think in terms of social class, it will nevertheless be important to build up a social-class profile of present and future clientele in order to plan promotional activities. Like it or not, this information can be extremely useful for predicting consumer behaviour, based on

- where clients live;
- their income;
- their education and occupation;
- their social status and prestige spending.

Note the needs of different groups, which can be classed as formal or informal, depending on their structure. For example, consider the characteristics of the family group or household. Its needs are based on:

- the earning capacity of the partners;
- their education and occupation;
- religion and lifestyle;
- who the decision maker is;
- the amount of leisure time.

## Psychographic segment

This can be used to build up a lifestyle and personality profile of a particular group, and to determine their buying attitudes and what benefits will be sought by extrapolating quantitative demographic, psychological and usage data.

This discussion is continued when we look at the client/hairdresser relationship and explore the client's perception of your standards (Chapter 4).

## What are the benefits of a market analysis?

A market analysis enables you to:

- assess present and future client concentrations;
- identify market opportunities;
- determine with a reasonable degree of accuracy how a niche market can be reached rather than firing indiscriminate shots into the dark hoping that one will land where you want it.

It is worth noting that it is not always the largest segment that is the most profitable. However, any segment can be profitable as long as you identify it, research it well and target its needs.

## Market segmentation summary

Assuming you have identified a client niche, the questions you will need to answer are:

*What:*

- are you offering?
- services do your clients require?
- benefits are sought?
- standard will your client expect?

*How:*

- will these potential clients hear about you?
- much should you charge?
- will you tailor your services?
- far will they travel?

☐    *Why:*

- do these clients buy?
- should these prospective clients buy from you?

☐    *Who:*

- are your competitors?
- buys your competitors' services and why?

## Get your figures together

In order to manage your future business and marketing strategy successfully, you will need to have a clear picture of your track record to date. This must show:

- how much money you have in your business;
- where the money in your business has come from;
- what the money was used for;
- your trading income to date;
- a breakdown of how the money you earned was spent;
- the level of your expected spending in the future;
- what your money will be spent on and when.

In simple financial terms this can be represented by the equation:

**Money in from clients – Money spent = Profit or loss**

This can be expressed graphically as follows:

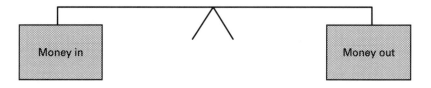

'Money in' represents income from fees for your services, product sales and any other sources of sales or revenue, such as training courses or promotional activities.

'Money out' represents the cost of sales which can be split into materials used in the salon for hairdressing plus your wages and salary bill including employer's national insurance contributions together with your running expenses.

A state of balance exists when Money in = Money out. If the money in is greater than the money out, you are in profit. However, if you have spent more than you have earned in any period of trading, you will be in a loss-making position.

To obtain a complete financial overview you will need to have and study the following accountancy documents:

- the balance sheet
- the profit-and-loss account;
- a cash-flow forecast.

Each will provide you with different information necessary for forward planning.

The balance sheet provides you with information on where the money in your business has come from and where it is currently used, i.e. funds, assets, loans and creditors.

The profit-and-loss account is a detailed historical record of how well you have done over a certain period.

A cash-flow forecast, as the name implies, is a forecast of when future income will be coming into the business, together with a schedule for planned spending each month over a set period.

These three documents can be used as management tools in the following ways.

The balance sheet enables you to know your current assets and liabilities if you have to restructure your borrowings or funding of the business.

The profit-and-loss account enables you to measure how well you have done over the period based on income earned (this is not the complete picture, however). It also means that you can identify where you have over- or under-spent as regards your outgoings. In addition the profit-and-loss account enables you to curb your future spending, i.e. to cut costs, and of course it makes it possible for you to identify whether you have made a profit or loss for that period.

By means of the cash-flow forecast you can structure your future spending, and time the payments each month to coincide with your estimation of projected monthly income. You will also be able to extrapolate important data including break-even point and gross and net profits.

You will now have a very good barometer for measuring how well you have done that will give you essential data for your future pricing strategy.

It is not within the scope of this book to offer a detailed treatment of how to prepare accounts. However, I hope you will follow through the overview in more detail and if necessary seek advice from an accountant.

## Pricing strategy

Pricing strategy should be based on:

- your past financial track record;
- the demand to date for your services;
- your fees to date for your services;
- what prices your markets will bear;
- how much your competition charges;
- a policy of dual pricing, where experienced stylists charge more for the same service than newly-qualified colleagues; prestige pricing, identifying the experienced stylists with prestige titles such as 'senior stylist manager' and charging to reflect this; and price cutting;
- increasing sales revenue to offset overheads;
- changing a client's perception of value;
- whether you can defend increasing your fees with improved quality or service.

## Market research

The sole purpose of market research is to reduce the area of uncertainty in the making of business decisions. It requires the collection of relevant data and information on present and future client needs.

What, how and where you collect the data and other information will depend on your objectives. These must be clearly established before embarking on such a project if you wish to obtain accurate results and to avoid wasting valuable time and money.

These are the stages of market research:

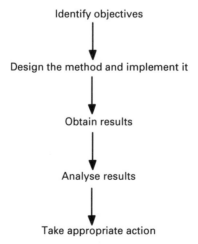

Identify objectives

↓

Design the method and implement it

↓

Obtain results

↓

Analyse results

↓

Take appropriate action

The usual reasons for carrying out research are:

- to get an idea of the size of the market in which you are at present operating or planning to do so;
- to learn about market prospects;
- to investigate how much your competition charges;
- to evaluate new services potential;
- to pinpoint the sources of client satisfaction;
- to find out more about the attitudes of your clients, i.e. why they buy from you in preference to your competitors, and how they heard about you; and to measure response to a sales promotion.

Market research: dig for data.

There are three sources of market research information that you will find extremely useful. These are as follows.

## Salon records

You will already have a wealth of information available including:

- client record cards (a must);
- daily appointment sheets or book;
- client bills;
- weekly and monthly sales-analysis records.

## Published information

You will be surprised how much free research information there is available from libraries, government departments, local council departments, trade associations and trade and consumer magazines.

## Clients

What better way to determine your clients' perception of value and your strengths and weaknesses than by asking customers directly by means of a questionnaire, or by asking them face to face or over the telephone.

# Taking your attack to the front line

So far I have outlined those marketing activities which take place behind the line. At some stage in the strategy the troops must be given the signal to advance. However, first the troops must be properly briefed with the tactics so they can carry the 'battle plan' to the enemy. The plan is to capture held territory and release those held captive and persuade them to come over to your side. This means giving them the choice that will enable them to make up their own mind. Before the advance, the area is targeted with leaflets with a message explaining the benefits to them.

You can employ a similar set of marketing activities to take your marketing plan to the front line. The tactics that you use are:

**Promotions:** A wide range of promotional activities can be used to persuade your target opportunities to leave your competitors and come over to your side.

**Personal selling:** This is a direct means of spearheading your advance to your clients through face-to-face communications.

## Promoting your business

Assuming you have targeted a specific client type, identified their needs, have a salon in the right location and are selling at a price that is affordable, you will not achieve many sales unless these prospective clients know about your services. You can have the best product in the world but unless you communicate this and put your message across, it may remain a secret.

Promotion is about communicating the key values of your business in order to strengthen your position in the market-place. Think: **the message, the market, the medium**.

Have you considered the following activities?

- Direct mail
- Exhibitions

- Sales literature
- Advertising
- Public relations
- Sales promotion
- Press relations
- Selling.

The three basic forms of communicating are written and visual, verbal, and non-verbal (body language). Whatever the method, it is important to consider carefully the stages of the communication process:

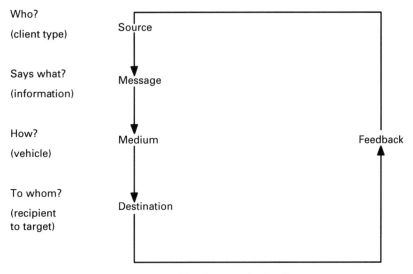

*The Communication Process*

## The message

This needs to be communicated in such a way that it first alerts the recipient to his or her needs, and secondly, indicates that you can meet these needs. People's attitudes are more easily influenced if information that they want is communicated clearly. You must know what determines client choice and the 'unique selling proposition' of your services.

## The market

*Who* are your clients?

◻   *What* facts and information on specific client types do you need to know in order to persuade them to buy your services?

◻   *How* will you reach your target audience; and what vehicles or media should you use to put your message across?

◻   *To whom?* You must get to know your potential target audience.

## The medium

If you were on a desert island hoping to find a way of being rescued, you might try putting a message in a bottle and throwing the bottle into the sea in the hope that somebody would read the message and take action. In reality the chances of this happening would be remote.

Once you have targeted your potential client audience and drafted the message, you need to be confident that it will reach them directly by the most successful and cost-effective route. The vehicles or media that are available to carry such promotional material are:

- business image;
- advertising in magazines and newspapers;
- advertorial;
- television;
- commercial radio;
- direct mail;
- posters and billboards;
- brochures and trade magazines;
- public relations;
- press relations.

Each vehicle has its own advantages and limitations. No one vehicle will reach all your potential clients regularly. So if you are planning a promotional campaign it is wise to choose a mix as part of your media plan that will suit your needs.

## Business image and design

### Think logo

A logo can be your name or a symbol or design that is used on all your stationery, literature, packaging, advertising, window signs, and any other design material to help clients to identify and remember you, your salon or group. Since it gets such wide exposure it is worth seeking advice from a graphic designer who is clued up on how to develop a corporate image.

## Briefing a designer

Commissioning artwork can be expensive. As always, you will get what you pay for. However, to save time and money and to appear professional, it is essential that you properly brief the designer with

- your objectives;
- a profile of the markets you are trying to target;
- what you want to use the stationery for;
- your budget for artwork and printing.

A rough visual may help to explain your ideas, and you should show the designer any photographic material that you have, and give them the copy that you wish to include. Now let the designer do the job of translating the brief into artwork. It will need to be proof read for mistakes before printing takes place.

## Preparing copy

Copy is the text that you wish to incorporate into your artwork. There is a skill in copywriting, and if you lack this skill you should pass on the task to a specialist copywriter.

## Think graphics

Graphics can be used to represent your services or product visually, using the power of print, photography, illustrations, layout, colour or black and white. They are best left to an expert who can translate your brief into artwork.

## From print to paper

With the advance in print and paper technology there are a wealth of alternatives to help you enhance your business image. Discuss them with your designer. Ask him or her about the following.

What will be the best typeface to use to enhance your style: is it upmarket or downmarket?

What will be the most suitable weight of paper? For example:

| business cards | 300 g |
| brochures | 200 g |
| letterheads | 110 g |

☐ The finish on the paper, smooth, matt, textured, satin, rough. Recycled paper doesn't mean cheap. What it sells is your awareness of the environment, which is very high on many people's list of priorities.

☐ Should the paper be laminated?

☐ Would it be better to use full colour if the budget allows, black and white, or tones of one colour (cheaper than full colour)?

## What's in a name?

Think this one out carefully. It is something you will have to live with for a long time, and besides it is important that you choose a name that is advantageous to your business image. Decide on a name that will be easily remembered, and one that flows off the tongue easily, especially over the telephone. Consider using:

- your own name;
- a composite name if you are in partnership;
- a descriptive name or phrase.

## The value of a business card

Small as they are, business cards are an essential piece of corporate stationery. A card can be used as a means of introducing yourself or as a calling card for future business opportunities. Measuring 8.5 cm × 5.5 cm, on average the basic card must be small enough to fit into somebody's wallet, 'Filofax' or record card system, and it needs to carry vital information:

- your company name and logo;
- the name of the person and position;
- the address and telephone number of your company, salon, etc., with clearly laid-out graphics on one side.

For a more sophisticated style of business card you may like to consider a double card folded. This will give you the opportunity of further promoting your services inside, and it can stand up freely. Another style of business card that is popular incorporates a small photographic image of, say, a product, a person or even a location.

For many people in the creative world of hair, make-up and fashion styling, who frequently need to promote their services to fashion or beauty editors, the larger format A5 size or Z card is most popular and will certainly give you ample space to include a sample photographic image of your work.

## Sales literature as a promotional tool

Of all the five senses the ones that are most crucial for businesses to get right are those that rely on impressions transmitted visually and orally. Very few of you will use radio, television or even marketing videos to communicate your message, but orally rely on either good telephone technique or face-to-face selling to promote your wares. However, on many occasions, even before we get a chance to 'sell' ourselves personally, we need to resort to other promotional tools such as sales literature. Think of the times when you have wanted more information about a company and what they offer. What do you do? You probably ring them up and ask them for more details. Such information can be effectively communicated using the power of graphics and copy contained on a flyer, in a brochure of even using a folder as a containing device.

Whatever you decide to use, think *visual*, think *style*, think *image*. In the hands of somebody who does not know you, it literally represents you on paper. Don't fall into the trap of designing a brochure to appeal to you yourself. It must appeal to your clients and prospective clients and their needs. They will be interested in the following:

☐ Your philosophy: what makes you stand out from the competition.

☐ The services you offer.

☐ The quality of your services.

☐ Where they can find you. A map of the location is useful.

☐ Your reputation ... even including client testimonials.

☐ A profile of you or details of your salon track record.

## Advertising your services

Advertising is another aspect of the overall promotional mix that relies on paying for putting 'print to paper' to communicate a message using a wide range of media such as magazines, newspapers, calendars, direct mail, directories, flyers, posters and gifts. The favourite media for many salons are the magazines, which offer advertising in the classified sections and the main body of the magazine, and in the form of what is called advertorial.

Whatever you choose, beware: it can be costly, particularly if you plan a series of advertisements. You must, therefore, define your objectives clearly. These may include the need:

- to target new clients;
- to target regular clients and interest them in more of the services you offer;
- to increase customer loyalty among regular clients;
- to counteract competition, either locally or nationally;
- to announce a particular service you offer;
- to maintain visual contact with the pubic;
- to boost your overall image;
- to persuade prospective clients that you are the company to do business with;
- to probe new market territories;
- to reinforce other aspects of your promotional campaign.

You must have a well drawn-up promotional strategy that takes into consideration:

- the market you wish to target;
- the message you wish to convey;
- how you are going to communicate the message graphically and verbally;
- which media you use;
- how much it will cost;
- how much you are prepared to spend;
- how you will monitor and measure the results.

To answer these questions you may well have to seek professional advice from an advertising agency, but at least do some initial research yourself. If you decide on using magazines, ask for their media pack. This will contain valuable statistical data on their reader profiles.

In our discussion on advertising, so far I have considered external advertising. Don't ignore the benefits of internal advertising, using professionally produced

- display cards
- photographic material

- leaflets or brochures
- posters

that enhance your internal salon image.

## Sales promotion

Like other promotional activities, sales promotion offers another means of increasing the demand for your services. It is a communication activity that can be used on its own or to supplement advertising and personal selling. In a competitive market-place, no high street these days is free from shops willing to offer discounts, for example on a particular product, on a holiday booking, at a restaurant or even when taking out insurance. Sales promotions go on throughout the year and are often geared to fall in line with seasonal influences such as Christmas, New Year and Easter, and to special events such as Mother's Day and Valentine's Day.

They are defined as a non-recurring activity, and their aim is a short-term one, namely to:

- provide a boost to sales;
- introduce a new product line;
- make your name more widely known, i.e. to increase brand awareness;
- reintroduce a product or service and hence to capture fresh interest, e.g. by offering a discount on a colour rinse;
- compete with Joe Bloggs round the corner who has set up in competition;
- introduce your services (by way of an introductory offer);
- capture new clients (by running a special incentive offer for a limited period);
- reduce stock levels of a product that is not selling;
- persuade former regular clients to return;
- move end-of-range stock ready for the new season;
- incentivize a purchase (by offering a free gift).

### Sales promotion and value

Ideally, sales promotions work best when they are set up to run for a limited period, providing a company with a vital boost to sales. However, at whose and what expense?

There is no value in setting up a promotion if:

- you have no clear objectives;
- it is not properly tailored to a particular market;
- it weakens your existing image by appearing tacky;
- the special offer is insignificant, i.e. has little value;
- a special prize is not prestigious;
- it is perceived by existing clients as gimmicky;
- you cannot meet the potential demand due to insufficient resources;
- the timing is not right.


## Planning a sales promotion

By now I'm sure you are fed up with hearing about developing a strategy. There's no point embarking on a sales promotion without first asking yourself these questions.

- What do you wish to promote?
- What do you plan to offer as an incentive?
- Will the area of coverage be local or national?
- Who are the targets, i.e. what is your market?
- How might they respond?
- What are your objectives for this activity?
- What will you call the promotion?
- When do you plan to run it? Is the timing right?
- How long do you intend to run it for?
- How will you promote it?
- Do you have the manpower to meet the potential demand, taking into consideration days off, holidays, sickness?
- Will the potential demand affect your regular clientele?
- Are your staff adequately trained to offer a service you wish to promote?
- Do you have sufficient stock levels to meet a demand for, say, a technical service?
- If you are giving away a free product, do you have sufficient supplies?
- Have all staff been consulted to enable you to hear their views?
- How much will it cost you to advertise it properly?
- Can you afford to give away mass discounts or other costly offers that may well affect your cash-flow forecast and profits?
- How are you going to measure the response?
- Have you taken into consideration such legal matters as 'special money off' and the requirements of the Trade Descriptions Act? Seek legal advice.

# Public relations

Public relations is a planned activity; its goal is to establish and improve effective communication between, say, an individual or organization and another party with the objective of assisting that individual or organization to enhance, build or retain a good reputation. 'Party' refers to another individual, a group of people, a company or an organization.

For a salon to improve and increase public awareness of its image and services, public relations is a relatively cost-effective means of promotion. However, it needs working at consistently.

One means at your disposal is using the power of the media to carry your message to the general public. The media can be radio and television, which rely on the speaker; or the press media such as magazines, newspapers and trade publications which rely on the written word supported by visuals. For most salons the latter will be the most fruitful vehicle to concentrate on. However, each relies on being fed good newsworthy items, features or 'stories' contained within a media document called a press release.

For little investment other than your time, if you have the flair to write, understand what it takes to write a good press release, and know who to contact, you may be lucky to land your press release face up on the desk of the news, features, beauty or fashion editor and not in the bin.

Developing press relations is an excellent way to get good editorial coverage. The essentials to writing a press release are that you:

- Come up with an 'angle', a newsworthy item about you or a business activity.
- Keep the words (copy) clear and concise – and interesting.
- Keep it to one side of headed A4 paper.
- Use double line spacing between the lines and have a 1–2 cm border surrounding the text.
- Include a contact name, address and telephone number, just in case further information is required.
- Indicate when the 'story' is to be released.
- Conclude the press release with the word 'end', centred about 1–2 cm below the final copy line.
- If you are sending photographs together with the copy, ensure that they are of good quality and are accompanied by relevant information such as 'caption', style details, technique, products used and credits. Colour slides are not always acceptable.
- Send the material in a clearly labelled cardboard envelope marked 'Please do not bend'.

## Monitoring response

There is no point, after investing time, money and human resources in planning and running a promotional activity, to let the response go unmeasured. How else can you evaluate whether it has been a success? If it hasn't, you will know that you should try a different approach next time.

Where better place to collect valuable response data than through your reception? Brief your reception staff to 'dig for data', either over the phone or in the salon when clients are making enquiries or placing bookings.

Devise a simple set of instructions and questions to ask as well as a form to record the information on. Once the promotion is finished, correlate the information before you are ready to draw conclusions.

There is no reason why monitoring should be confined to promotional activities. Use similar techniques to build up a weekly profile of the clients you serviced that week. This will give you information on:

- how many regular clients;
- how many referral clients;
- how many new clients;
- those clients who receive a discount;
- any compliments and complaints;
- how many clients purchased products;
- the clients who buy specific services;
- your peak booking periods.

This information will be very useful when it comes to making an inventory on your business sales to date.

## The final assault

Before I focus attention on the key marketing activity in our industry, selling, and the person who delivers the service as well as the interaction with the clients, I want to stress the need to have a battle plan.

Your battle plan is a formidable weapon against the 'enemy', competition. Your marketing plan should contain your marketing concept in detail. That is, all the marketing activities that will help you to identify and satisfy clients' needs must be welded together in a logical, coherent document which in turn must be part of the overall plans for your business.

## Your marketing plan

For explanation see accompanying notes.

### Developing a Marketing Plan

Stages                                           Questions to Ask

Diagnosis            (1)                 Where are you?

Prognosis            (2)                 Where are you going?

Objectives ———→(3)                       Where do you want to be going?

Strategy (4)    Budget (6)               Have you analysed the market
                                         opportunity and your company's ability?
                                         What resources will you require?

Tactics (5)◄————————┘                    What marketing activities will suit your
                                         objectives? Who will carry them out and
                                         when?

Control (7)                              How can you check that your objectives
                                         are being achieved?

Points                                   Notes

(1)    Analysis or inventory of the present position of your business, leading
       to a statement of its problems.
(2)    Establishing priorities.
(3)    Setting goals that you wish to accomplish during the marketing time
       period. The objectives need to be qualified quantitatively as well.
(4)    Analysis of your target opportunities and your company's resources,
       e.g. manpower, financial, equipment, training, promotional material,
       needed to achieve your goals.
(5)    Your action plan stating what has to be done in terms of marketing
       activities: who will carry them out and in what time period.
(6)    Allocating and organizing sufficient funds to accomplish your goals.
(7)    Planning and applying a feedback system to monitor the results.

# 2
# The Art of Selling

## The hairdresser versus the salesperson

So far we have established that marketing is a concept devoted to planning how to make your services available to clients who need and want them. We have established that in order to promote your services you have a number of processes to choose. One such process that I will be concentrating on throughout the book is selling.

For some reason the word 'selling' seems to many hairdressers to invite an unfavourable response. I remember my early days as a junior stylist when it was a weekly practice to call each stylist into the manager's office to discuss their sales figures from the previous week, only to be told that you were not meeting your client targets, departmental referrals and product sales targets. Yes, you knew that if you 'cut' more clients or talked them into having colouring, perming or purchasing haircare products, your commission would be better. We worked hard, played hard. Little responsibility meant poor commitment. Lack of commitment meant little regard for how much money we earned, as long as we could get by. As far as many were concerned, we were artists, not sales people, our sole aim being to reach the pinnacle of perfection in our work.

It was fine if a client asked if she could have a tint, a treatment or buy a bottle of shampoo, but we would not go out of our way to suggest buying one. Suggesting meant having to talk money, a dirty and difficult word for many to discuss.

As I became more established, my responsibilities grew and I soon realized the importance of making a decent living to sustain my lifestyle. Making money became more important. It was at this time that I began to refocus my thoughts on selling, thanks to an inspired training programme I attended called 'The Art of Selling'.

Day One started by talking about the difference between a goal and a purpose. The trainer then told us that it was important for everybody to have goals, something that one can accomplish, whereas a purpose is more ongoing and gives meaning to one's life. Having a purpose is fundamental to your enjoyment of everything you do ... how good it makes you feel.

The trainer then asked for a show of hands in response to the following questions:

'Who finds it difficult or uncomfortable to adopt the role of a salesman?' All hands went up.
'Who finds it difficult or uncomfortable to speak about money to their clients?' All hands went up.
'Who agrees that earning money is important to sustain one's standard of living?' Again all hands went up.
'Who would like to have more fun, enjoy your work, be less self-conscious about selling to clients, still earn money for your services and give the clients what they want?' All hands shot up.

The trainer then showed the following on an overhead projector:

YOUR MOST IMPORTANT GOAL IS TO CREATE AND KEEP CLIENTS.
- Forget about trying to get what you want but start helping your clients to get what they want and need.
- Help them to buy what's best for them.
- Make them feel good about it.

He went on to explain that there is a big difference between selling and helping clients to buy:

Selling creates a sale whilst helping people to buy creates customers. Forget the manipulative approach to selling: let's change your attitude.

He continued:

Find out what the clients want and need, and see if you can help them; be it through your services or products. Make it your purpose to help your clients get those good feelings they want about what they have 'bought' and about themselves (see Part II, The Relationship).

Money, although still a goal, now becomes a natural by-product of your main purpose. Clients *hate* to be sold but love to buy, especially if they know what you are offering is going to make them look younger, more attractive, more confident.... It's all about *caring* about your clients.

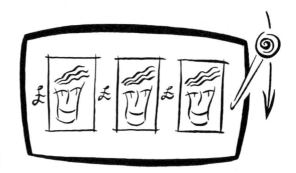

You're a winner too!

By the afternoon of the training programme my attitude towards my work, clients and employer had changed. I could see that a professional hairdresser needed to be both a salesperson and an artist. It made sense: how else was I to present and promote my ideas and skills? Sales are simply a way of communicating them.

I left Day One feeling excited and that I had been given an amazing insight into what makes a successful hairdresser. The trainer showed that you need to be

- a motivator
- an effective listener
- a persuasive communicator
- a subtle closer (see The Consultation).

But how was I to apply this knowledge? Perhaps this would be explained on Day Two.

## The anatomy of a sell

I arrived for Day Two excited in anticipation of what was to follow. The theme for the morning session was 'How to reach your objective by applying the four elements of sale'.

The trainer began by writing on the flip chart the letters '**AIDA**'. 'Does anyone know what they stand for?', he asked. There was silence for a while and then he continued.

The answer is:

"**A**" is for attention,
"**I**" is for interest,

"**D**" is for desire,
"**A**" is for action.'

Remember this: it will help you give structure and flow to your sales.
First you need to capture your client's attention, as shown, and then follow through with stages 2–4.

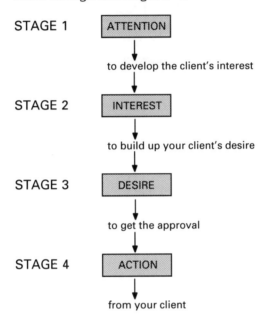

STAGE 1    ATTENTION

to develop the client's interest

STAGE 2    INTEREST

to build up your client's desire

STAGE 3    DESIRE

to get the approval

STAGE 4    ACTION

from your client

## How to help your clients to buy your services

These four stages will help form the foundations of your initial consultation skills. Although these are the starting point for finding out more about client needs, they also provide an ideal opportunity to promote your services, products, etc.

Let us now look at the different stages of AIDA more closely and see how they work.

### Attention

Needless to say, you must be confident of capturing the client's attention from the first moment of contact (see Part III, Marketing Yourself), and maintain it constantly throughout your sales pitch. To do this you must communicate in terms that are relevant to the client, who wants to know what's in it for them.

This is achieved by

■ getting your clients or potential customers to communicate areas of interest; and then by
■ personalizing their needs to suit their lifestyle, personality, etc. in terms of benefits to them.

Clients buy benefits, not features. Features are particular aspects of your haircuts that come through your technical and artistic expertise. What your client buys is what it can do for them, in other words, provide solutions to their problems.

## Link words

Use key words in your sell to link features to benefits: 'this means that ... because ...'.

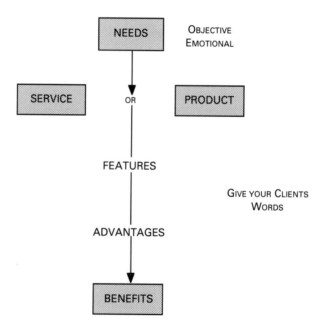

## Benefits and needs

It's no use coming up with a list of the benefits that, say, a restyle is going to achieve if they are not relevant to your client's needs. Benefits have to be viewed as the solution to a real need which they are conscious of . . . or can be made to be conscious of.

Your clients' needs may be of two kinds: those that are objective and rational and those that are emotional and sometimes irrational. Clients will be motivated by both types, but it will be only the objective, rational kind that they will be prepared to acknowledge.

## Objective/rational needs

A client who is interested in a hair restyle may hope that it will:

- take off the split ends
- make their hair look thicker
- make it easier to manage
- save time in the morning
- be more versatile.

## Emotional needs

Clients' emotional needs lead them to hope that a restyle will:

- give them more confidence
- make them more attractive to their partner
- make them look and feel younger
- improve their career prospects
- enable them to catch the eye of the opposite sex.

It is your job to find out what their true motives are, to establish which are the most important, and then to emphasize the benefits accordingly.

This is a time for tact and sensitivity (see Chapter 3, 'The Confidence Factor'). Few clients volunteer this sort of information; most would like to let you believe their decisions are solely rational. However, the more experienced you become, the more will you be able to 'read between the lines'.

It is essential to make the link between your clients' needs and the benefits as clear as possible. For example, two different clients may visit your salon for a colour but expect it to do quite different things for them, for example hide their grey hair, create greater impact, or enhance face shape and features. They are each looking for different benefits. It's down to you to assess each client's problems. This I will discuss more fully in Part IV.

## Interest

Interest and attention are very closely linked. Attention is what is gained by your basic proposals; interest is what is aroused and maintained by the facts that you put in front of your client in support of your argument.

### *Techniques*

▨    A client will respond favourably if they feel you are well focused on their problem.

> CLIENT:    I have extremely dry hair.
>
> HAIRDRESSER:    I certainly agree with your need to repair your damaged hair. I would suggest you have a protein reconstruction treatment to help make your hair more shiny and easier to style.

Here the client will be impressed to find that you are interested, you have listened to them, you understand their needs, and you can save them time.

▨    Clients will respond favourably to sincerity and truth.

> HAIRDRESSER    May I recommend you buy these products to take home with you. They will help you to care for your hair in between salon visits.
>
> HAIRDRESSER:    Although the products may seem initially more expensive than others, they are the best for your hair condition. You will only need to use a very small amount as they are very concentrated. If you use an amount each time the size of a pea, each bottle will last you $x$ months. This means you will save money in the long term.

▨    Clients will be interested if you come up with ideas or can suggest an alternative way of meeting their needs.

> HAIRDRESSER:    Have you considered . . .?

▨    Use colourful words to excite.

> HAIRDRESSER:    The colour will add *richness* and *vibrance* to your natural hair colour.

▨    Be aware of your body language. Besides answering verbally use the power of positive expressions, mannerisms and gestures to say 'yes'.

▨    Use link words 'This means . . .', 'This is because . . .', to link features to benefits.

▨    Use the client's name and make sure you use the words 'you' and 'your'.

This draws the client's attention to what you are saying and helps them to feel more a part of the selling process.

☐    Show authority.

## Desire

Your aim is to keep the selling process running so smoothly that you bring the benefits and needs so close together in the client's mind that it sparks the gap and the sale is made.

Remember: you are appealing to a client's needs. You will know when you have succeeded in convincing your client to buy your services or products when they

- approve of what you are saying;

- ask you questions, indicating that they are listening to your recommendations;

- make statements indicating that they want to hear more.

- show positive body language signals.

## Action

'Action' means that moment at which your client agrees to your recommended services before being whisked off to the backwash, or wants to buy the products you have recommended to them.

In Part IV I will be applying the theoretical aspects of making a sale to the very practical foundations of 'interpreting your clients' needs', starting with the consultation.

# PART II
# THE RELATIONSHIP

# 3
# *The Confidence Factor*

## Why do clients visit the hairdresser?

Have you ever asked yourself why clients visit the hairdresser? Although this may seem an obvious question, it is extremely complex and is heavily influenced by a variety of needs including the desire:

- to receive a new hair image;
- to seek professional, objective advice about how they look;
- to get reassurance and build self-confidence;
- to be kept up to date on beauty and fashion trends;
- to be able to talk to somebody who will simply listen to their problems;
- to socialize;
- to obtain sanctuary at least for a few hours in a place where they can be themselves and be totally pampered.

Whatever their motives, clients do not buy what you or your salon sells. Instead they buy what your services or products can do for them.

## A love affair

The best way to describe hairdressing is to say it is a love affair: with the profession, a belief in yourself, your skills, products, and the service you offer, combined with a love affair for (notice I did not say *with*) your clients.

According to journalist Kimberly Leston:

The secret for the perfect haircut is a journey at least as profound as any quest for a grail ever was, filled with danger, yet rich in rewards for those brave enough to face their true selves . . .

Most women are obsessed with their hair in some way because no-one is ever really happy with it. In the end it is the longest love/hate relationship any woman ever has. The personal success or otherwise of your relationship with your clients will depend upon:

- whether you can come up with solutions to their problems;
- your ability to make them feel good about their actions and about themselves;
- how good you feel about yourself (see Chapter 6, 'The Real You').

According to behavioural psychologists a person is capable of experiencing only four basic emotions, the feelings of being glad, sad, mad or scared.

Clients only buy when they are feeling glad about you and your services. It's a question of winning their trust and of giving them confidence in themselves.

The confidence you give to your clients will depend on whether you show them how involved and identified you wish to be with their needs in contrast to your desire to assert your individuality (see Chapter 8, 'The Elements of Style').

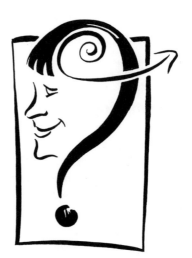

Glad, sad, mad or scared?

We all have these needs within our make-up. We express them through our appearance, how we speak and our body language. However, often they clash, registering conflict with others and disharmony with ourselves.

# Your relationship style

When cementing any relationship with someone new, you need to work to develop your relationship style. For the relationship to have true value, you need to decide the extent to which you play the following roles.

(1)  Do you act as a good friend to your client and play a *supporting* role?

(2)  Do you take the part of the adviser and play a more *informative* role?

(3)  Do you take the part of the critic and *confront* the client? (I hope not).

The key is to maintain a balance of (1) and (2) with a small amount of (3). This balance can be represented as follows:

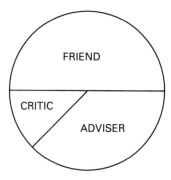

Part of the secret of the success of this relationship lies in understanding your clients' feelings and in recognizing their emotional needs.

# Feelings and emotions

How many times have you heard somebody say, 'I've got something on my mind'. What do they mean? Where is the mind? How does it work?

The mind is a large reservoir of knowledge within your brain. The brain works like a biological computer into which all our knowledge and experiences are fed and filed away for future reference. As well as controlling our mechanisms, thoughts, feelings and responses, the brain acts as a data bank, processing the information until such time as we need to react to messages relayed to the relevant parts of our body.

Our feelings involve a chemical chain reaction in our bodies. Certain chemicals are released into the bloodstream, according to the emotional reaction stimulated by your thinking. Consider those times in your life when you have experienced such feelings as love, joy, anger, anxiety, fear or sympathy and how they influenced your behaviour.

Four basic emotions

| Glad | Sad | Mad | Scared |
|------|------|------|--------|
| Love | Sympathy | Anger | Fear |
| Joy | Depression | Hate | Nervousness |
| Happiness | Anxiety | Fight | Apprehension |
| Security | Unhappiness | Motivation | |

Your clients will also experience such feelings but each will have their own emotional make-up and different problems that need to be solved. Their decisions to buy are based on unconscious needs and wants, such as habit, prestige or perceived value (see Chapter 4, 'A Client's Perception of your Standards'). Few will acknowledge that they are responding to emotional reasons for buying.

The key to winning and keeping clients is to respond to each client's wants and problems, and by helping them to like themselves better.

Any successful relationship or partnership calls for a high level of collaboration from both parties. The client has an important part to play in the relationship and has to be encouraged by you to 'play the game'.

Winning is not beating the client into submission so they have what you want. Instead you can both win: the client gets what they want, you get what you want (another satisfied client).

## What is confidence?

Confidence comes from within. It reflects a balance between being happy and unhappy. It is very much a product of our state of mind. We are all affected by our level of confidence. It can transform our lives, depending how much one has in reserve. It is the key to our well being and self-fulfilment, to the possession of a positive outlook and to having a

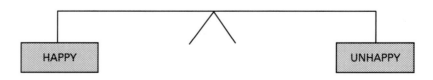

contented life. To achieve the right balance takes precise adjustments, especially at different stages in our lives.

You might say 'What has this got to do with hair?' My answer is, 'A great deal'. It is important to remember that you are dealing directly with clients' emotions, their needs, and levels of self-confidence. This can be a combination of their

- Self image: what sort of person they think they are;
- Self-esteem: how good they feel about themselves;
- Body image: how good they feel about their body.

## Understanding a client's emotional make-up

How many times have you heard a client say, 'I hate looking at myself in the mirror'? This is a feeling that has probably arisen over a period of years during which they have developed a cumulative assessment of what they look like, usually arising out of their relationships with family and friends who make comments and suggestions or give advice on how they look or should look. Typical comments include the following:

'You always look scruffy.'
'Your hair always looks a mess.'
'You have a big nose like your father.'
'Grey hair really makes you look old.'

It is therefore no surprise if they have little confidence in how they look. Body image does not necessarily have a lot to do with body shape. A client may think they are overweight, too short or too tall even though their proportions are perfect.

Many clients develop a 'conceptual image' of how they think they

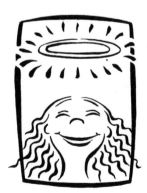

Body image: I'm OK!

should look that again has been built up throughout their childhood, into adolescence and then into adulthood. Much of this can be attributed to cultural and media influences or the prejudices of others. Also, when they look in the mirror, there is a conflict with their perception of the ideal body, which is not that of a real person.

Others may well be going through change in their lives. For example, they may be having to readjust to major upheavals such as divorce, bereavement, unemployment or illness. These are all factors that can contribute to low self-esteem.

In a relationship in which the partners have changed at a different rate and in different ways over the years, a confidence problem can often arise if either is heavily discouraged from changing the way they look. A classic example of this is the middle-aged woman with long, naturally grey hair who says, 'My husband likes me with long hair'. What she is saying is, 'I am not confident to make decisions to suit my needs and am too heavily influenced by others.'

Unfortunately, a partner or friend cannot be totally objective. Their vision is too influenced by their own prejudices, experiences and stereotypes, and is full of emotional attachment. For example, most men assume that long hair on a woman looks sexier, and would usually object to their having it cut shorter even if it was more flattering.

Whatever the reason, learn to 'read between the lines' and watch for the telltale signs of a loss of confidence, particularly with those clients whom you have known for some time. Probe very gently.

## Telltale signs

- An increase in weight and general lack of interest in their overall grooming.
- A loss of weight can also indicate a body image problem.
- Hiding behind a curtain of hair.
- Talking with the hand over the mouth.
- Walking with the head bent forward.
- No social life.
- Negative star qualities (see Chapter 5, Selling Yourself).
- Mood swings.

Through understanding and reassurance you can help them to overcome their problems, or at least work towards helping them to look more attractive. It's amazing how looking great can give a person a tremendous boost of self-confidence. Be well satisfied when you hear a client say, 'My hair looks great, I feel like a new person.'

# A positive attitude

Some years later when I was in a management role, I began to notice a developing trend: it wasn't always the most artistic hairdresser who had the largest clientele. I started to look for possible reasons for this. Before I consider these, I would like to describe the time I was standing near to reception, observing how it was operating. A customer approached the desk and asked one of the receptionists if she could get some advice on improving her hair condition as well as ideas for a restyle. On taking the customer through to the consultation area the receptionist proceeded to use the internal intercom to buzz downstairs to the staff room for a stylist to come and speak to the customer. After about ten minutes and following a further request, a stylist sluggishly appeared and went through to speak to the customer.

From where I was standing I could see and hear their interaction. I was embarrassed and annoyed at the lack of enthusiasm, passion and time that the stylist gave to the customer. I was most surprised: he was one of the salon's best cutters. It was hardly surprising that the client soon got up and began to walk towards the salon entrance. Attempting to rescue the situation, I approached the customer, introduced myself, apologized for the attitude of my stylist and asked, 'Do you mind if I help you?' She agreed.

I proceeded to explain what would suit her best and would improve her hair condition, and to discuss our other hairdressing services. Before long she had made an appointment to come in for a total transformation.

Has this happened in your salon? It illustrates one of the fundamental principles of selling:

- clients can be persuaded more by the strength of your beliefs and emotions than by any amount of logic or knowledge you possess. It's a question of attitude.

It is essential that you remember two important points about client behaviour:

- Clients are ruled by their emotions, how they feel.
- Emotions are contagious.

Clients don't care how much you know about hair or the products you use *until* they know how much you:

- care about them as people;
- believe in your services and products.

# Confidence boosters

Every client wants and needs to have their confidence boosted or affirmed. Focus on building your client's self image. Help them to like themselves better and you are well on the way to making a positive and lasting impression. If you damage the client's self-confidence, you're in for a hard time. You will make it easier on yourself if you understand that clients only buy when they feel glad about you and your services.

## *Techniques that work*

- Practise the 'art of good conversation' by getting clients to talk freely about themselves. Listen with your undivided attention. Already they will feel better.

- Praise your clients. Every person likes a compliment or to feel that they have made the right decision.

  > 'You look at least ten years younger.'
  > 'Your new style really enhances your bone structure.'
  > 'Your new eye make-up brings out the colour in your eyes.'

- Put your star qualities to work. Remember laughter and good humour can be a great tonic for a client who is feeling low.

- Practise good body language and make them feel relaxed, at ease and not threatened ((see the section on body language in Chapter 8).

- Help them to visualize how good they could look. Often the thought of change may not be so bad after all. Use carefully chosen words and visuals if necessary to help describe an image.

- Many clients need constant reassurance that they have made the right decision. Use logical reasons to convince them.

- Use good communication skills to problem solve by moving clients from a mad, sad or scared state into a glad state (see Part III).

  > 'Is there any aspect about your hairstyle that you unhappy with?'
  > 'How do you finally visualize your new hairstyle?'

- Work on balancing your appearance to be appropriate for the salon and type of clients you deal with (see Chapter 8, 'The Elements of Style').

# 4
# A Client's Perception of Your Standards

## Your business image

When it comes to promotion, knowing Who, What, How and Whom is essential, but there is no point getting these communication stages right if you are to be finally let down by how your message is perceived. This introduces the important area of business image, the face that your company/salon presents to its customers. It is how clients perceive you and the impressions which are formed.

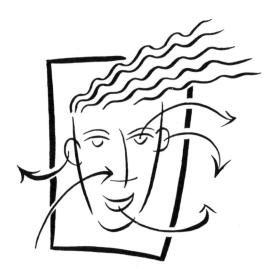

Impressions.

As the book develops you will understand that my philosophy on business image encompasses the **quality culture** of the business, made up of the external and internal face of the organization, and the image presented by personnel at all levels. This is the **total image concept** (TIC) of an organization. Applied to salon situations, it is the sum total of all the perceptions your clients and all others have about you, your staff and the salon(s).

Every business needs an image. It requires careful planning, hard work and consistency to ensure that all the areas work in harmony with one another and reinforce company objectives.

TOTAL IMAGE CONCEPT

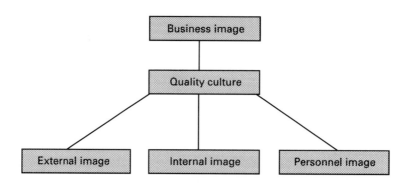

Image is established, maintained or improved by the standards you set, that is, through the following inputs:

- the quality of your hairdressing services;
- the way you go about delivering those services;
- the quality of the interpersonal relationships with your clients;
- the design image of the salon;
- your corporate identity.

STANDARDS AS A BAROMETER OF QUALITY

The quality of inputs will influence the clients' perception of your business

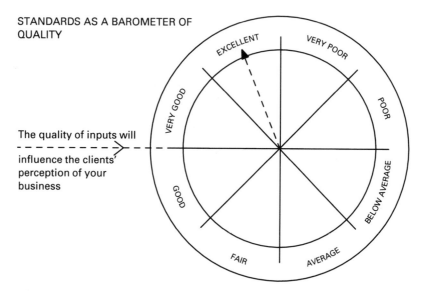

Standards are rather like a barometer, falling, staying constant or rising according to the quality of the input. The input means the elements, features and characteristics which contribute towards your total business image.

Standards can be defined as a level of excellence or proficiency, and are measurable and attainable.

# A total business image checklist

## External image

- Name
- Logo
- Business stationery
- Sales literature
- Advertising
- Sales promotions
- Public relations
- Salon location
- Neighbours

- Pavement area
- Shop front
- Signs and fascia
- Window display
- Entrance
- Telephone sales
- Days open
- Hours of trading

## Internal image

### Interior design

- Salon layout
- Decor
- Furniture and furnishings
- Equipment
- Flooring
- Lighting

### Environment

- Comfort
- Air conditioning
- Ventilation
- Music
- Noise
- Atmosphere
- Conversation

### Domestics

- Hygiene
- Tidiness
- Cleanliness

### Service resources and facilities

- Products
- Refreshments
- Towels and gowns
- Toilets and changing room
- Reception waiting area

### Internal advertising

- Photographic

- Sales literature
- Signs
- Display material
- Packaging

## Hairdressing skills

- Shampooing
- Cutting
- Blowdrying
- Styling
- Dressing
- Conditioning
- Colouring
- Perming
- Retailing

## Service delivery

- Consultation skills
- Reception system
- Telephone technique
- Waiting time
- Service delivery time
- Manpower
- Interpersonal skills

## Personnel image

- Star quality
- Appearance
- Grooming
- Communication
- Vocal image
- Body language

# Standards of excellence

I recall the story told to me by a friend about a male colleague of hers who wanted to buy a new car. He and his wife were attracted to an advertisement in their local paper and decided to pay the garage a visit one Saturday afternoon. They drove on to the forecourt of the garage. As soon as they had parked and got out of their car, they were greeted by a salesman who shouted, in an abrupt, aggressive manner from the other end of the forecourt, 'Move that car over there'.

On getting back into their car, the husband turned to his wife and said, as they drove away from the garage, 'That guy's just lost himself a sale. We'll go to that other garage across the road.'

This incident is a typical example of the increasing and rightful intolerance customers have these days to indifferent service, shoddy workmanship, faulty goods and other activities or actions that do little to create a positive impression. In an economic environment in which suppliers are competing for customers, many now recognize the potential of quality as a secret weapon in the world of business management. Standards of attainment of both the service and service-delivery characteristics are being clearly defined, and can be evaluated by the service organization and customer in order to bring about greater customer satisfaction.

There was no excuse for the car salesman's rudeness and poor service. Hairdressing is no different. It too is a service industry. It makes no difference whether you are dealing with a new or a regular client; each deserves respect and attention, and calls for customization of your services.

Whether the client is having a shampoo, a restyle, a blowdry or a technical service, a great deal of faith and trust will be placed in you. For many a visit to a salon will be magic or misery. Many clients visiting a salon for the first time find the experience intimidating, especially if they lack self-confidence (see Chapter 3, The Confidence Factor). Every time you come into contact with a client they will come away feeling better or worse about their experience – hopefully better. It is down to you to perform the service with a clear understanding of what it takes to create and keep clients.

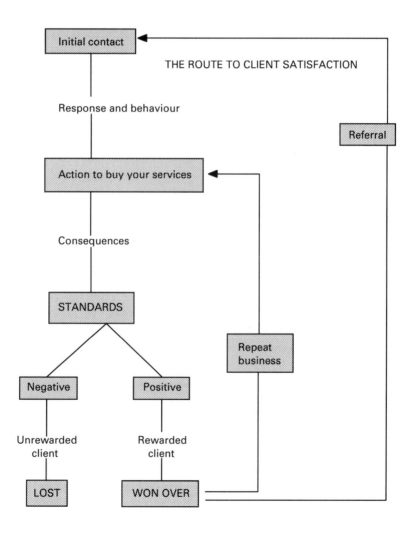

The difference between successful and profitable salons and the unsuccessful ones will hinge on their standards of excellence in filling the needs of their customers. Working at achieving client satisfaction is therefore far too important to leave just to the owner or manager of your salon It should concern *everyone* from within the salon or group.

It is no secret that client-focused management should be sensitive to trends and changes. The factor that distinguishes the successful from the unsuccessful business is the ability of management to grasp the principles of building a quality culture. This culture must be based on a well formulated quality policy of clear intentions, objectives and directions for the salon to operate under. A philosophy of quality management must be followed in which everyone understands, implements and maintains a quality system. In such a system, responsibilities, procedures and resources for implementing quality management within the salon must be planned carefully.

Staff should not be excluded from contributing to quality management. However, essentially the lead must come from management. Each manager will have his or her own style and winning formula. Success will not be due to any one element of that formula but to the delivery of services to each client in an integrated and balanced way. The success stories have one thing in common. That is, that clients want to buy their services and keep coming back.

## What makes a quality system?

Unlike a manufacturing business, where the customer is rarely or never seen, in a service industry such as hairdressing, you and client meet face to face. The meeting point at which the product changes hands is known as the interface.

A hairdressing salon may seem a relatively simple service operation. However, that's until one looks more closely into its mechanics and realizes that:

- it is manufacturing a product;
- it demands the management of the interface (the client relationship);
- it consists of multiple interfaces, i.e. receptionists, apprentices, stylists, manager.

An interface can be split into two parts, the production interface, where the service is 'manufactured', and the delivery interface, where inter-action with the client occurs. In a hairdressing operation, although there will be different delivery interfaces (the reception area, the backwash area, the technical department and possibly a beauty area) by far the most important production interface is the styling position.

In a manufacturing industry, a factory, say, the delivery interface occupies only a small proportion of the total operational area:

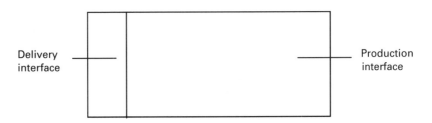

Delivery interface ——————— Production interface

In a salon the delivery interface occupies a greater proportion of that area:

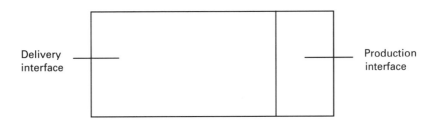

Delivery interface ——————— Production interface

The critical factors in hairdressing are:

■ Managing the production interface (the standard of work);
■ Managing the delivery interface (the standard of services);
■ Getting right the balance between the two.

## Key players and the team

If you are part of a team, when you are dealing with a client you are the company to that client and their decision to become or remain a client depends on *you*. You will be judged not only on how you deliver the service at your respective interface (your work skills) but also, and equally important, on how you market or sell yourself.

I have used 'marketing' in a much wider sense here to introduce the important concept of self-presentation which I will be developing later.

Depending on your size of operation, the members of the team can be represented traditionally by a **Team Tree**.

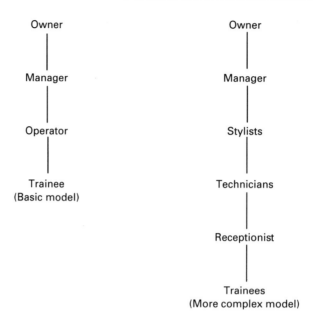

Now turn these trees upside down.

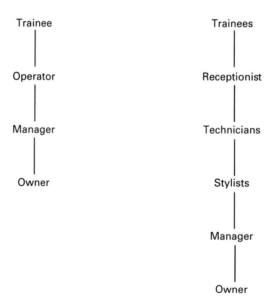

I do this to illustrate the point that although there is no doubt a degree of hierarchy in your salon, if you are a team member, no matter what your position within your salon or company, you have a vital contribution to make. You are a vital link, a key player.

Now form the tree into a circle and put the clients into the centre.

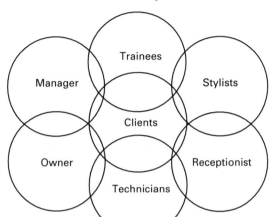

The salon will still be judged by:

- both positive and negative impressions
- the general atmosphere
- how smoothly the different interfaces operate
- the overall team mechanics
- but *especially* by how client-centred the team is.

A *client-centred team* is one that is:

- well focused on client needs
- supportive of each other's needs
- hungry for a good performance
- able to generate ideas
- given clear performance standards
- united and happy
- clear about team objectives
- well balanced
- able to communicate with each other
- rewarded for its efforts.

In such a team there is little room for weak links.

## Quality management overview

If you are a manager or supervisor, the team will look to you for leadership qualities. If you are the salon owner, the team will expect management direction, security and reward. You will become a figure-head.

It is appreciated that in many cases the owner and manager will be one and the same, and that the size of the team will vary according to the nature of your operation or group of operations. The logistics become more complicated when the organization grows and there is a need to operate with a management team. In a sense the members of such a team have propelled themselves to the top through their own personal achievements and sense of individualism, which may conspire against team behaviours. This makes teams at the top a difficult entity, although this will depend on how they in turn are managed.

The successful management team concentrates on the following important aspects:

- securing the stability of the business through adequate resources, i.e. financial and manpower;
- working at building, maintaining and continuously improving a quality system;
- developing a harmonious relationship between team players and with clients.

Key factors of a quality system

Note: The client is the focal point of a quality system.

# Quality control

No team can be asked to perform well without clear guidance as to what is expected. No machinery can be expected to run smoothly without regular servicing of the infrastructure. It is a function of creative management:

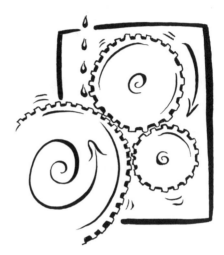

Quality control: lubricating the mechanics.

## To plan:

- how each service can best be delivered to the client;
- what system to use to achieve the task;
- how to deploy manpower effectively and efficiently;
- how to use technology;
- effective support for the team infrastructure;
- how systems can be improved.

## To motivate by

- communicating a vision of the future;
- setting performance standards;
- providing clear and realistic objectives;
- stimulating individuals to set their own goals;
- leading by example;
- instilling confidence;
- working with the team in setting standards.

## *To reward by:*

- showing appreciation;
- recognition and praise;
- setting team incentives;
- providing job security;
- fairness;
- loyalty.

## *To communicate. This means:*

- opening up two-way communication with clients;
- registering and recording feedback from clients;
- passing on feedback to the team;
- holding regular dialogue, both informal and formal, with the team to discuss performance;
- holding annual interviews with team members aimed at playing a supporting role;
- asking the team about their needs;
- encouraging ideas and suggestions to flow;
- holding brainstorming sessions with the team.

## *To supervise:*

- monitoring how well the team performs;
- monitoring how each team player contributes;
- walking the job (you cannot supervise from an office);
- identifying any problems that are disrupting team performance.

## *To train:*

- through a commitment to developing others;
- holding regular coaching sessions;
- implementing a team development programme;
- encouraging an atmosphere of learning;
- helping members to develop an understanding and appreciation of each other's jobs.

## *To finance by:*

- ensuring that there are adequate funds to cover business activities in the short and long term;

- setting prices for services;
- monitoring and recording transactions;
- controlling expenses.

## To act:

- decisively and fairly;
- by taking tough decisions even if they may be unpopular at the time;
- by being willing to make changes happen;
- by responding to feedback;
- by settling any disagreements or conflicts which will undoubtedly arise from time to time;
- by listening openly to team matters.

## To care:

- through support;
- through loyalty;
- by guidance;
- with friendship;
- and by boosting the self-esteem of every member of staff.

If a person feels good about themselves they will produce good results.

## Teamwork breakdown

A breakdown in teamwork will undoubtedly result in:

- the fine balance of the team being upset;
- poor overall performance;
- a drop in standards;
- unfair workload on motivated members;
- eventually a fall in sales.

This can be brought about by

- poor recruitment;
- an individual team member's dissatisfaction;
- poor team spirit;
- unclear objectives;
- directives or company policies that are out of date or have not been well thought out;

- weak communication from management;
- poor communication between team players;
- lack of support between team players;
- insufficient job motivation;
- lack of recognition, reward or other incentives;
- failure to provide essential equipment and technology;
- faulty equipment;
- inadequate training and career development;
- an ineffective quality control system or one that is not implemented;
- a lack of ideas;
- management with tunnel vision.

## The shaping of impressions

Before I look at this exceptionally important issue, I want to introduce the idea of perception by using colour as an analogy.

Colour is an integral part of our everyday lives: we explore it from an early age, we use it, perhaps without really questioning it or appreciating the powerful effect it has on our lives or on others. Such is the power of colour that throughout history it has been the subject of great fascination for artists, poets, scientists and philosophers.

Colour is an energy, a vibration, with the power to relax, excite, stimulate, sedate. Different colours are known to have a 'nutritional' value and to have the potential to effect subtle chemical changes within our bodies.

Colour has been used throughout time to convey our emotions and experiences. Used aesthetically, colour can transform one's environment. Applied to one's physical appearance, colour can be used to attract, to convey the right impression and to boost the wearer's self-confidence. Used wrongly it can diminish one's appeal.

I'm sure you have your favourite colours as well as those that you dislike. What is it that attracts or repels us about particular colours? Our response to certain colours is a complex physiological and psychological relationship made up of visual images or stereotypes based on emotional and physical experiences stored in our memory. The response is influenced by:

- religious beliefs
- cultural values
- society values
- our prejudices

- our associations
- superstitions
- symbolic meanings.

All these result from experiences in our childhood, adolescence and adulthood. Our aesthetic beliefs, how flattering we think certain colours of clothes, make-up and hair are, can also be influenced by such social pressures as the media, advertising and idolization of role models.

Evidence from scientific research suggests that light of different colours entering the eye can affect specialized regions of the brain which control our expression of emotion.

# What our senses tell us

You are probably saying to yourself 'What's emotion got to do with a client's perception of me and the services I provide?'

Clients respond to any visual images that can be used to communicate or transmit a message, be it the design of the salon, advertisements, brochures or business cards through to your appearance or that of other salon personnel. Clients' response to these different sources and the subconscious actions they may take will be shaped by their values and beliefs, based on their physical and emotional make-up, past experiences, stereotyping and irrational prejudices. These irrational prejudices can result in a barrier being formed between you and your clients, so hampering your ability to communicate effectively.

How initially impressed clients are and whether they form a lasting good impression will depend on how the images are received.

- Eighty-five per cent of what we remember comes through seeing.

- Eleven per cent of what we remember comes through hearing.

  We can also be favourably impressed if we hear and register something that appeals to our sense of values and beliefs, so it is understandable why client recommendations are so effective.

- Our senses of touch, smell and taste also play a key role in registering things we like. These account for the remaining four per cent.

  No matter what the size of your salon, you rely on good reputation and quality service to get clients to come back. But are these sufficient?

  You may be dedicated, staff may be well motivated, you may spend time planning how to serve your clients well, *but* until you make your

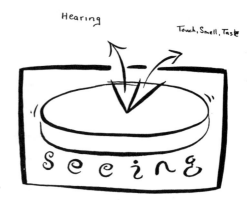

Sensing: what our senses tell us.

clients feel that you are customizing your services especially for them and that they are getting their money's worth, you will have an uphill slog.

It's not the quality of service that you give your clients but the quality of service that they perceive which encourages them to buy your services and come back. This may sound strange but it is essential to remember that:

Perceived service quality is the difference between what your clients get and what they expect.

It's as simple as whether service is perceived as good or bad; what their expectations are and whether they are made to feel glad, sad or mad.

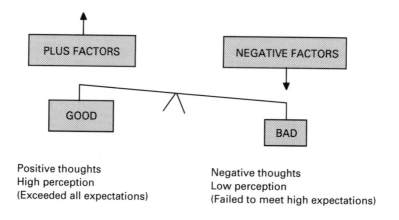

Positive thoughts
High perception
(Exceeded all expectations)

Negative thoughts
Low perception
(Failed to meet high expectations)

The more plus factors, the greater the left scale tilts upwards, increasing client perception and hence client satisfaction.

Pay attention to even the smallest detail. It is often this that impresses the client the most.

## Can you be totally objective?

So you think you are doing OK – but are you? How you see yourself and how you want others to see you may not be how clients really perceive you. Wrapped up in this statement is the argument that it is not always possible to be truly objective about your services.

☐ Your judgements may be based on false values and prejudices.

☐ Being unfairly critical of other hairdressing establishments may well obscure a realistic assessment of the competition.

☐ You may be too close to your business to view it objectively. You may be being over-passionate about your operation, which can give you blinkered vision.

## How to improve a client's perception

As I explained early on in the book, every business has and needs an image. The image of your salon influences how clients perceive the environment they are sitting in, the people that surround them, and the manner in which they are served and by whom. Leaving it to chance is a sure recipe for failure. There is no substitute for careful planning, starting by building up a client profile of the clients you want to win over (see Part I, Developing Your Client Marketing).

The more clearly you can define which customer types you are trying to reach and serve, the easier it will be to perceive your business through their eyes. Equally, it is important to perceive your business through the eyes of your existing clientele. Do this by taking stock, educating clients, and through client feedback.

### Taking stock

Imagine you are a client in your salon. Begin by evaluating the following.

*Look* at the:

- Staff's appearance.
- Salon design.
- Colour scheme.
- Furniture.
- Equipment.
- Product displays.

- Photographic material.
- Flooring.
- Corporate literature.
- Magazines.
- Flowers.
- Cleanliness.
- Tidiness.
- The standard of work.
- Non-verbal communication.

*Listen* to the:

- Telephone technique.
- Conversation between staff and clients.
- Conversation between staff members.
- The appropriateness of music.

*Smell* is also important, so note the many aromas that waft around such as chemicals, smoke and smells that relate to personal hygiene.

Finally, *taste* the quality of the refreshments served, and *touch* the work surfaces, product displays and gowns.

Would you be suitably impressed? If not, what can you do about it?

Take as an example the basic selling technique market traders use to sell their products. They will always tell you what great value you are getting by buying from them. Selling your services is no different. It's not enough to reward your clients with good service: you have to make them aware of the great value they are getting.

## Positive impressions

Here are some ways of creating that vital favourable impression.

- An accessible location.
- Prominent exterior design and front window display.
- Attractive, well groomed personnel.
- A good standard of dress.
- Attractive decor, with an eye for colour coordination and colour harmony.
- High standards of cleanliness and tidiness.
- Flattering lighting.
- Regular refurbishment.
- Up-to-date equipment.

- Comfortable seating.
- Good ventilation.
- Comfortable room temperature.
- Well presented photographic material.
- Professional looking artwork on stationery, sales literature and advertisements.
- Concise and grammatically correct copy.
- Eye-catching product displays.
- Up-to-date magazines.
- Clean gowns and towels.
- Fresh flowers.
- Well served refreshments.
- Not charging for refreshments (all inclusive price).
- Staff playing the perfect host or hostess.
- Good service at a fair price.
- Client contact: updates, newsletters. Building on client recommendations.
- Consistency and care.
- Punctuality and good time-keeping.
- A reception area that functions effectively.
- Telephones that are answered speedily.
- A knowledgeable receptionist.
- Good telephone manner.
- An efficient booking system.
- A welcoming smile.
- Friendly, helpful professionals in all areas.
- Quality professional skills.
- Zeal appeal. A1 for effort.

## Negative impressions

Negative impressions are created through:

- Poorly groomed and turned-out personnel.
- A poorly maintained salon.
- Badly chipped paintwork and marked walls.
- Unattractive decor.
- Ineffective ventilation, leading to condensation on windows.
- Uncomfortable room temperatures: too hot or too cold.
- Unswept floors.
- Broken light bulbs.
- Dirty styling positions and chairs.
- Empty product displays.

- Tacky work surfaces.
- Dead flowers or plants.
- Plastic plants.
- Dusty surfaces.
- Dirty towels or gowns.
- Musty smelling towels or other abnormal smells.
- Badly torn towels.
- Dirty brushes and combs.
- Stained or chipped crockery.
- Torn or tatty magazines.
- Faulty plumbing.
- No toilet paper in the toilets.
- Poor hygiene of both personnel and salon.
- Clients being kept waiting.
- Clients being let down at the last minute.
- A dictatorial attitude: 'Have what I say . . .'.
- Arrogance (an attitude problem).
- Unhelpfulness and lack of courtesy.
- Lack of social graces.
- Staff talking over client.
- Promising what you can't deliver, i.e. not coming up with the goods.
- Unsuitable music.
- Staff chewing gum.
- A lack of after-care service.
- A hard sell.
- Bad language.
- Shouting across the salon.
- Staff arguing.
- Sexual harassment.
- Always asking regular clients to produce their cheque card.
- Impolite form of address.
- No change at reception.
- Mistakes in the bookings.
- Low prices may give the impression to some clients that the service is of a lower standard.

## Educating clients

You may know that what you offer is special, but do your clients? You may be the keeper of the world's best kept secret, your services. They will remain a secret unless you bring them to the client's attention and explain:

- your product mix;
- what benefit each service will bring to clients;
- what excellent value they are;
- why they are special;
- their features.

## Client feedback

If you are in business to please, you cannot start to make improvements in the management of your standards until you know how your services are perceived by clients. To win clients you must constantly look at ways to provide a better and better service.

I'm sure you have been out with a partner, friends or family to a restaurant and left very disappointed about the poor standard of cuisine or the service. But did you complain? Instead, you probably paid the bill and vowed never to go back. Very few of us take the trouble to either telephone or write in with our complaints, comments or suggestions on how to improve a system, and very few businesses bother to ask.

My strategy for improving the quality of services and service delivery is an *outside-in* approach to client-centred marketing which involves communicating directly with one's clients to clearly define true values. The truth may hurt, but failure to find out how you could do better is very short-sighted and a sure way to lose valuable repeat and referral business.

Measure client satisfaction by using the following methods.

### Design a written questionnaire

This must:

- be brief, and ask specific questions about your standards;
- use well thought out, open-ended and closed questions;
- include a rating system based on a scale from, say, 1 to 8, where 1 is excellent, 2 is very good, 3 is good, 4 is fair, 5 is average, 6 is below average, 7 is poor, 8 is very poor;
- be designed to extract useful market research data;
- sample sufficient clients to make it worth while.

The best time to use a questionnaire is while the client is in the salon. At least this way you can be sure of getting a reply back, whereas postal questionnaires require prepaid envelopes which will bump up the costs. Furthermore, can you be sure of getting them back? You may wish to target ex-clients and find out why they haven't been back.

Once you have collected the data, it's up to you to process it quickly, interpret the results objectively with team members and act to enhance your services. Repeat this cycle of feedback at a later date to remeasure results.

### Random sampling

Use the technique of random sampling by targeting, say, 12 clients each week just before they leave. Ask them if they could spare a few moments to answer a short service questionnaire verbally. Offer them something for their trouble.

### Client suggestions book

Keep this at reception with a notice asking clients to record their impressions and suggestions for improving your salon services.

### Client representative sessions

As part of a client-centred approach to quality management, hold regular sessions for a small group of invited clients to discuss salon services openly.

It is important to note that such feedback may

- contain biased answers;
- be too small in sample numbers to give a realistic picture of your total clientele;
- be unspecific because you have asked the wrong questions.

### Telephone after-sales

Go one step further down the quality route by introducing an after-sales support service, especially for those clients who may have had a major restyle or technical service.

## Dealing with an angry client

I can vividly remember the one occasion at the beginning of my career when I met head on with an angry client of mine. She had the right to be angry. It was a Saturday – those appointments every 15 minutes were dreadful: for the client who was expected to wait, and for the hairdresser who had to cope with irate clients. I had two choices, either to be helpful or to take a defensive stance. You've guessed it, I chose the wrong one.

Instead of being apologetic I retaliated to the irate client's verbal abuse. Needless to say, it didn't help. For the entire time the client was in the chair, I was the centre of her fury.

It's not a mistake I would make again. Here is my advice on how to deal with an irate client. Start by applying a little bit of sound psychology. Instead of making the client even more annoyed, work on their feelings by passifying their anger. Convert their emotions from a state of feeling mad into a more happy state by:

☐ Remaining cool, calm and collected even under pressure. This is essential. On no account attempt to argue: if you do, you will have to face the consequences.

☐ Watch your body language too: don't take up a defensive position.

☐ Listen carefully to their criticisms. This will help you to come up with positive solutions later. Avoid taking the criticism personally. Once an angry client realizes you are interested and they have been made to feel you really care, you are on the way to winning them over. As you listen, use positive facial expressions plus lots of empathy and nod your head to say non-verbally 'Tell me more'. (see Chapter 8, Body Language)

☐ Next, respond to their comments by sympathizing. For example:

'I can quite understand how you feel about being kept waiting . . .'
'I fully appreciate your annoyance about having coffee spilt over you . . .'
'I completely sympathise with you about having your booking messed up . . .'.

If it was your own fault, apologize profusely. If you are acting on behalf of the salon and you know that, say, a staff member was at fault, again apologize.

☐ If you still need to seek further information, ask suitable questions:

'I can see you are annoyed, but can you tell me who was rude to you?'

☐ Once you have a good grasp of the situation, move decisively to take positive action to appease the client. You may like to offer, as a gesture of good will, a number of options for the client to choose from, such as a free treatment, a complimentary service next time, or a refund.

# Dealing with complaints

No organization welcomes complaints, but those that have initiated a policy of resolving customer dissatisfaction by developing a complaints procedure will be rewarded for their investment in quality management. Good can come out of complaints, for the following reasons:

☐ They can give you a measure of how well you are doing, where possible weaknesses may be in your system and where improvements can be made. Don't think of a complaint as negative feedback: treat each complaint positively.

☐ It is not often one is given a second chance to rectify a poor service and improve client satisfaction. Be grateful to the client for taking the trouble to complain. Just think of those clients who don't bother – and who don't come back.

☐ It will give you the opportunity to convert a complaining client into a loyal client, especially if you retrieve the situation through your resolve to win over the client.

Most complaints in a salon are likely to be due to a poor standard of workmanship or an indifferent service. Whatever the reason, do everything to reward complaints with speedy, positive action.

## Tips for handling a client complaint

Many of the skills for dealing with a complaint I have covered in the previous section. Here is a summary of my recommendations.

☐ Stay cool.

☐ Do not react defensively, verbally or non-verbally.

☐ Listen with empathy and interest to the nature of the complaint.

☐ Sympathize . . . and apologize.

☐ Don't blame others or make excuses. What's happened is history to the client. All they will be concerned with is what solutions you can come up with.

☐ Speed is the essence.

▨   To ensure you have grasped an important point, use a paraphrasing technique to repeat it back to the client.

> CLIENT:   I distinctly said I only wanted to have only the split ends trimmed.
>
> MANAGEMENT:   Let me make sure I fully understand . . . you specifically asked for a trim. Is that correct?

▨   Show your concern and willingness to help by using appropriate body language (see the section on body language in Chapter 8).

Deal with complaints before clients leave the salon. At least this way you can diffuse the situation and prevent the person spreading bad publicity. Often clients will not complain to their hairdresser, but will do so when they are paying their bill. Brief the reception staff to report a complaint, however small, immediately. Discuss with your staff the salon's philosophy on the handling of complaints as part of your programme of continuous improvement and your strategy for ensuring customer loyalty.

If a client sends in a complaint letter, you will need to reply promptly, either offering some form of compensation or preferably requesting they make an appointment to come back to the salon so that the complaint can be processed. It will help if you have a complaints form to record essential information, namely:

- the client's name, address and telephone number;
- the name of the operator or persons involved;
- the date of the original appointment;
- how much they paid;
- the nature of the complaint;
- action taken or to be taken;
- guidelines for improvement;
- date of follow-up;
- further action if needed.

If you need to go and speak with another person or check out a piece of vital information, excuse yourself and tell the client you will be back in a moment. Make sure that if they are left they have magazines or refreshments.

At this stage you will need to find out what the client wants.

> MANAGEMENT:   Once again, Mrs Smith, I would like to say how very sorry I am about the service and I would like to propose that we:

- Give you a discount.
- Offer you a refund.
- Offer a complimentary haircut in 6–8 weeks.
- Redo your hair right now.
- Look after your hair free of charge for the next *x* months until you are fully happy.
- Give you a course of complimentary hair treatments.
- Give you this 'goodie' bag of haircare products free of charge.

Make sure the level of solution matches the nature of the complaint.

Be decisive in your offer of settlement. Bring the complaint to a conclusion by asking the client if they are happy with your solution. Hopefully, they will be. If not, why not? If they are simply being unreasonable and you are locked in a stalemate, or if you feel they complain for the sheer sake of complaining, you might be better to give them a refund to save wasting any more of your time and politely excuse yourself, especially if you have left your own client to attend to the complaint.

Make a courtesy follow-up call at a later date to see that the client is still fully satisfied. This also drives home your customer care policy.

If during any stage of the procedure you are unable to 'problem solve' a solution, seek advice or authority from your line manager.

# What to do if you realize a client is going to be disappointed

This in essence encourages you to take the initiative if a service has not been performed well by yourself or a member of staff. You must bring the problem to their attention first, before they find out for themselves. Whilst the client will be initially disappointed and may be upset, your policy of being honest will certainly enhance your client relationship and pre-empt an otherwise angry complaint later. Attempting to hide or deceive the client is asking for trouble.

For example, a client may rightly be disappointed if:

- you realise a client's hair is still greasy and continue blowdrying;
- a colour has not taken properly or a perm has an uneven curl;
- you misinterpreted their hair type and texture and the style has not worked as well as you expected;
- there has been a misunderstanding;

- there has been a human error;
- the client's expectations were too high and they came down to reality with a big thud!

Whatever the reason, the client is naturally going to feel let down. Your job now is to handle the situation with sensitivity and restore their confidence by:

- First apologizing.
- Alter the tone of your voice to convey your apologies.
- If you get aggressive, you're likely to have an angry client to deal with.
- If it was due to a misunderstanding, don't say to the client, 'I thought you knew what I was going to do.'
- If the client is disappointed because of failure to meet their high expectations, don't say to the client, 'What did you expect? I'm not a magician.'
- Coming up with positive solutions to put the matter right, as quickly as possible. The client does not want to hear excuses or hear you pass the buck, run down a colleague or blame it on the product. They come to you because you are the professional. To restore your professional credibility, behave in a professional way.

To come up with positive solutions you may need to reactivate your consultation skills and find out where a breakdown in communication occurred. Agree with the client on what action they would like you to take, before you proceed.

The lesson to learn for next time is:

Prevention is better than cure.

# PART III
# MARKETING YOURSELF

# 5
# *Selling Yourself*

## Your total image

Meeting people of all types from all walks of life is part of your everyday life. How they warm to you, what vibes you give, how others receive them, how well you win them over and conversely how they appeal to you are the very essence of forming successful relationships whether at work or socially.

How you both 'gel' is an automatic process, an intuitive sixth sense initiated by how you both interpret each other's signals received and controlled by your own respective computer systems, the brain. This acts as a data bank, registering and recording one's daily experiences, evaluating them against expectations and beliefs, before initiating a response in the form of an action to be taken.

From that initial meeting, depending upon the intensity and frequency of the signals and how they are received, *attention* can be turned into *interest* and interest into *desire* to know more and hence to listen more attentively before deciding to take *action*.

What are these signals? They are made up of those magic ingredients called **star quality** or **charisma**.

## Star quality

Star quality is the magnetic attraction created by a delicate balance of signals transmitted by one person and received subconsciously by another. In the case of your relationship with clients, although you can attract on different levels, intellectually, emotionally or physically, these signals are most effective when they are the result of your total image, how you:

- look
- stand
- express yourself
- think
- project your beliefs
- feel
- behave.

They contribute greatly to how well you sell yourself to others (your projected image) and how others perceive you (your received image).

<u>A Model of How You Sell Yourself To Others</u>

FIRST IMPRESSIONS

Your presentation ───────────────── A client's perception

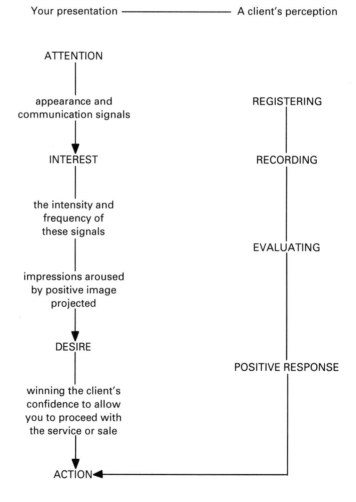

ATTENTION

appearance and                                  REGISTERING
communication signals

INTEREST                                        RECORDING

the intensity and
frequency of
these signals

                                                EVALUATING

impressions aroused
by positive image
projected

DESIRE

                                                POSITIVE RESPONSE

winning the client's
confidence to allow
you to proceed with
the service or sale

ACTION◄─────────────────────────

Don't for one moment underestimate the qualities you need to have to become a complete hairdresser. No longer should hairdressing be viewed as the career for the less able. Its demands are many and the rewards great, and a good standard of education combined with enthusiasm are important. There is no one ingredient that a successful hairdresser needs, but a blend of many: that magic ingredient called star quality, and the skills that come from experience and formal training.

I'm sure you have all met, heard and been in the company of individuals who hold your attention with their personal magnetism, charm and winning personality. We instantly identify this mysterious something as star quality or charisma.

Charismatic individuals are found in every walk of life, from public figures to entertainers, from politicians to spiritual leaders, from actors to pop stars, and even hairdressers. You seek out and look up to such people. You learn to respect and admire them for their qualities. Some people have more star qualities and hence greater charisma than others.

What does star quality really mean? Recognizing someone with star quality is an emotional reaction in which we respond intensely to those individuals who touch our innermost emotional selves. Such people may have special qualities including:

- Self-motivation
- Vitality
- Courage
- Composure
- Warmth
- Sincerity
- Receptiveness
- Sensitivity
- Compassion
- Intelligence
- Leadership
- A positive self-image.

Other characteristics that increase our perception of a person as having star quality are:

- Status
- Wealth
- Talent
- Beauty
- Humour
- Attractive appearance
- Accent
- Articulacy
- Sense of fun
- Fame
- Expressive facial language
- Expressive body language

The greater the characteristic the more are we attracted to the individual. Stars are by definition individuals.

Think of the individuals you know. What attracts you to them? What star qualities do they have?

## Clients buy star quality

Combine the following ingredients plus your other star qualities and you get what it takes to satisfy a client's needs.

### Empathy

This is the ability to understand your client's opinions and feelings without necessarily sharing them. This is not the same as sympathy, which involves sharing the client's feelings. Put yourself in their situation.

### Enthusiasm

Enthusiasm is contagious. It will help to stimulate your client, attract attention, arouse interest, give confidence and lay the foundations for a successful sell. It is important to gear the level of enthusiasm to every client's needs.

### The ability to listen

Listening and empathy combined are essential qualities to help you discover what the client really wants (see Chapter 9, on listening).

### Alertness

Reinforce your listening skills by being able to understand what clients are saying by their body language.

### Integrity

Having a reputation for honesty is a most valuable quality.

### Loyalty

Never run down your colleagues, boss or any other member of your salon in front of a client. Total loyalty to the salon or company, salon management and even the product is essential in order to create a good business impression.

### Reliability

You must give your clients what they want each time to the same standard of excellence, i.e. you must be consistent.

## Responsiveness

You must respond to a client's needs as quickly as possible, without keeping them waiting.

## Tolerance

This means understanding that clients may have opinions that differ from yours, and respecting those opinions.

## Acceptability

Display appropriateness of dress, grooming and behaviour to reflect the company/salon image.

## Belief in yourself

You must have a firm belief that your work is of great value.

## Resilience

You must be able to perform well even when you are unwell or having an off day.

## Credibility

You must be able to give your clients peace of mind, and convince them that you have their best interests at heart.

## Politeness and courtesy

Use the correct mode of address.


# Meeting a client for the first time

When clients meet you for the first time, they begin by checking out your image signals, looking for subtle clues, evaluating them against the data bank of information that they have on people. Their assessment of you is made up of visual images or stereotypes and is based not on a single element of your presentation but on the total picture. The elements in that picture include:

- colouring
- gender
- age
- height
- facial expression
- eye contact
- hair and make-up
- build
- clothes and accessories
- posture and movement.

Your body is rather like a shop window. An empty shop window or one badly displayed will not attract any potential customers. However, if there are goods in the window suitably displayed, it might entice customers into the shop to look around, perhaps with a view to buying.

Similarly, our unadorned bodies cannot signal ideological differences so we turn to:

- clothing
- accessories
- hair
- make-up
- jewellery
- perfumes.

These and other suitable visual props together with non-verbal behavioural signals are used in an attempt to communicate the right messages about who we are and what we have to offer. The signals become a form of self-advertising which gives even complete strangers a means of communicating with each other.

In much the same way our response is a measure of the importance we place on packaging. Compare how we attempt to package ourselves and the packaging of a product. We are attracted to the size, shape, and colour but we still need to know what benefits are in it for us. It is often up to the salesperson to continue to arouse our interest by their sales pitch which gives us details of the benefits and uses the features of the product as supporting evidence to convince us to buy.

How you dress, the colour of your clothes, how you wear your hair, together with your overall grooming, all give clues or first impressions to others, revealing much about you, your:

- age
- lifestyle

- personality
- occupation
- sexuality
- political and religious beliefs
- inner emotions.

This is eloquently summed up by James Lever in his book *Style in Costume* where he describes clothes as 'the furniture of the mind made visible'.

## The need to impress

The elements that make up your total image are how you are judged. It can take as little as 30 seconds for somebody to form a lasting opinion of you. It is therefore of utmost importance during those initial moments to create a good impression. Such assessments are often unfair, yet appearance is the only means others have to judge you.

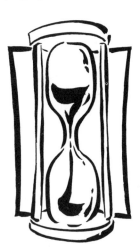

Create a good impression: the first few minutes.

We are told 'Don't judge a book by its cover', but we are all guilty of doing this. Rationally we know that the way a person presents themselves, their outer image, may not do justice to their inner image. Yet we still make those instant judgements of one another, and base on them our decisions as to how to start and continue communications.

Once people's interest has been aroused by our outer image, they have a desire to know us better. They come to appreciate our inner image or qualities, so our physical appearance often becomes less important.

According to behavioural studies by psychologist Albert Mehrabian, of those first impressions:

☐　Fifty-five per cent is based on what we *see*. This includes colouring, physical appearance, posture, facial expressions, eye contact and body language.

☐　Thirty-eight per cent is based on what we *hear*. This includes the tone, pitch, pace and clarity of a person's voice as well as the accent used.

☐　The remaining seven per cent is based on the *words* we hear.

We are able to form impressions so quickly when our impressions include character traits that fit a certain stereotype. We make the assumption that other traits that we have not yet seen will also fit that same stereotype.

# The element of style

We say 'That person's got style', but what do we mean? A lucky few are blessed with natural style. However, for most it doesn't come that easily. But what is style? Style is about attitude. Stylish people know themselves well enough to be themselves. Style is a reflection of who you are.

People who have style have one characteristic in common: confidence. Style reflects self-confidence to express their individuality in whatever they wear, their hairstyle and make-up, their poise, their presence, in fact every aspect of their presentation. At this stage we need to define the difference between style and fashion.

Fashion is very much what is current in the shops, is seen often in the latest magazines and is generally worn like a uniform by dedicated followers. In contrast, the stylish person creatively adopts fashion to enhance their physique, personality, age and lifestyle.

It is often said that one needs a lot of money to be stylish. Money may well buy the most expensive designer clothes and accessories but that does not necessarily give one a passport to looking great.

Looking good and presenting a polished image are not about vanity nor are they a question of ego; they are about an attitude to making the most of yourself, and self-improvement is essential for personal development. Attitude is what your clients will be looking for. Since you are in the business of making people look good and feel good about themselves, clients will tend to judge your ability on the basis of your looks, poise, presence and presentation. Your clients will be more easily convinced about your competence from the outset if they perceive that you share their beliefs, values, attributes and behaviour.

We tend to associate positive attributes with positive attributes and conversely negative attributes with negative ones. This is what behavioural psychologists refer to as the 'halo effect'. Thus, if your appearance and manner appeal to your clients, they are likely to assume that you are competent.

Let me explain this by asking you to imagine you are a client. You decide to get advice on your hair. You seek out two hairdressers. Hairdresser 1 has a very poor chairside manner, and hairdresser 2 has a good chairside manner. On the basis of this you make the assumption that hairdresser 2 is more technically and creatively competent than hairdresser 1 because the latter does not relate to you as well as the former. You want to be right and hope you are right. Only time will tell.

Another 'impression trap' that you need to be aware of is the tendency to think that people who are like us will think and behave in the same way that we do. The 'likeness effect' may first work in your favour, but make sure you can live up to their image of you. Similarly, just because you work in a salon with other hairdressers, all with a common interest, do not automatically assume they will all approach the job as you would.

Give your clients precise information to go on.

Wrapped up in these arguments is the question, 'How accurate are clients' impressions?' Much has to do with how they assimilate stereotypes and the associations they make. If their experience of life is limited or clouded with prejudice, then their irrational attitudes may go against you.

## Looks do matter

To this day the stereotyping 'what is beautiful is good' still exists, supported by numerous research experiments and studies on physical attraction, which established that attractive people tend to be happier, more successful, more content, more helped, more trusted, sensitive, interesting, more just about everything desirable. And even when they are not, they are perceived by others to be so.

Truth is not always reality but what clients perceive is reality.

As the saying goes, 'Beauty is in the eye of the beholder'. Whether we like to admit it or even realize it, we all judge people initially by how they look.

Looks, according to psychologist Dr Mayon Tysoe, '. . . do matter, we think that beautiful people have beautiful souls'.

It was the Greek poet Sappho in about 612 BC who said,

'What is beautiful is good
And who is good will soon be beautiful'.

So what is it that we are looking for? Who and what do we find attractive? To understand why we discriminate as we do over looks is outside the scope of this book. Suffice it to say that our perception of attractiveness is determined by our view of the perfect body, what we consider to be the perfect face shape, and matters of cultural upbringing, social changes, fashion trends, the media and gender signals.

A study by psychologists Wilson and Nias found that people's perception of attractiveness is based on the following characteristics:

- a great smile
- clear skin
- a healthy glow
- shining hair
- flattering clothes
- high self-esteem.

In reality personal attraction is more than simply appearance and physique: it encompasses one's entire total image and the elements of style.

## 6
## *The Real You*

## Your personality

In our daily lives we meet and look up to people who win us over. We seek out those people who possess special qualities: intelligence, perhaps, or sex appeal, personal style or a sense of fun and adventure.

It would be boring if everyone was the same. Thankfully no two people are alike. Their features are different, and they smile, laugh, talk, act and behave differently. It is therefore fair to assume that each has different qualities that set them apart. Such qualities express our individuality and are a major force in signalling first impressions to others. These qualities are your personality. Your personality is you. It reflects your self-image. Your level of emotionality can be expressed in terms of two personality types, who approach and experience life from opposite directions. The types are the extrovert and the introvert. Your image and how you present yourself will also be influenced by the levels of extroversion or introversion in your personality.

The **extrovert** is often perceived as:

- outgoing
- friendly
- expressive
- sociable
- energetic
- competitive
- keen at communicating their message
- welcoming stimulation from others
- one who works hard at being liked
- excitable.

In contrast the **introvert** is often considered to be:

- quieter
- more reserved
- less sociable
- calmer
- more stable
- often opinionated
- often a loner.

# Expressing personality

Your personality is expressed not only by what you do but by the way you do it. Non-verbal signals such as what you wear, how you wear it, hairstyle, overall grooming, facial expression and body language are the silent communicators, and together with the tone of your voice can reveal much about the kind of person you are.

Here are some different forms of expressive behaviours shown by the extrovert and introvert.

## The extrovert

The extrovert desires involvement and identification with others by:

- Wearing medium to deep contrasting or bright colours that explode with energy in the hope that they will attract attention.
- Making a fashion statement through a more flamboyant style of dress.
- Using more positive, expressive, facial expressions to show their emotions.
- Using more eye contact, especially during face-to-face communication.
- Moving the head more.
- Using the hands more expressively in gesturing away from the body; this conveys a relaxed, confident, warm and embracing personality.
- Using the technique of moving closer towards somebody and orientating the body towards them.
- The more frequent use of touch.
- Talking a great deal, often in an excited manner.
- Firing questions to seek involvement.
- Speaking with a firm tone of voice.

## The introvert

Introverts are very much preoccupied with their personal achievements and have little desire to seek involvement with others. They tend to:

- Attach little importance to wearing clothes that attract attention from others.
- Wear colours that are quieter, softer and less bold.
- Wear uncomplicated styles.
- Have little or non-exaggerated facial expression.
- Avoid eye contact.
- Make restrained gestures.
- Display more closed body language.
- Offer little touching or body contact.
- Converse economically.
- Take time to deliberate on vocal content, i.e. what they are saying.
- Speak in a soft voice.
- Like humour which is mainly intellectual and defensive.

Hans Eysenck has argued that, rather than fit people neatly into definite categories, it is more logical to locate people on continuous dimensions since we all have a combination of both extrovert and introvert tendencies, influenced by our genetic make-up, how we grew up and in what sort of environment, the people in our lives, and the situations and occasions we find ourselves in.

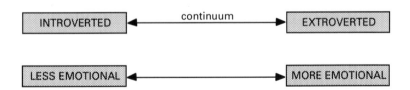

There is always a balance in the well adjusted person, although one will be more dominant than the other.

# 7
# Self-presentation

## Be your own PR

Earlier in the book I spoke briefly about public relations (PR) in a general way. I described it as the ability to increase public awareness of your business and put it across. It is selling to them. It is getting them to think highly of you. It is grabbing their attention, making them aware of your existence.

Large companies invest millions of pounds planning elaborate campaigns to launch new products or services or to change public opinion on existing activities. It is often very difficult to measure the results of a PR campaign whereas you can monitor the results of advertising and show a return on investment in terms of extra sales.

For our purposes we can reduce PR to a simpler level. In straightforward terms public relations is about presenting yourself, your company and your services in a favourable way to the general public, who will include regular clients as well as potential new ones.

You can be your own public relations man or woman by appreciating that a large part of the service you provide is 'showbiz'.

## You're on stage

Service delivery is like a theatrical performance. Are you or your staff adequately prepared for the star role? When the client is in the chair, you're on stage and the spotlight is on you.

Compare your performance to that of an actor or actress. It makes no difference whether they are appearing in a one-person show or a large production: each needs to prepare adequately before they go on stage. They do this by:

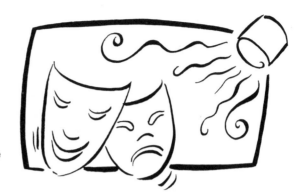

You're on stage: the
spotlight is on you!

- learning the script (i.e. the role);
- rehearsing how best to project the role;
- choosing whatever props such as wigs, false pieces, stage make-up and theatrical costuming are necessary to enhance the appearance;
- studying accent, tone and other elements of vocal communication before seeking to convince the audience about the role they are playing.

In our urban society 'acting' in the presentation of self is all part of the game of life. It often demands subtle changes to be made to our total image according to the script. By 'script' I mean the different situations, occasions, company and roles in which you are likely to find yourself during the course of work and play. You might need to evaluate the script and decide how best to play it to project certain qualities.

It is unlikely that you will go to the lengths to which actors go prior to performing, but you can prepare yourself very adequately for your 'performance' by looking to those elements of style – your wardrobe (clothes and accessories), appearance, good grooming, body language and verbal communication – to create the right impression.

In your everyday life, social acquaintances are established and relationships are formed by using the first impression as a 'filtering device'. New contacts undergo a social selection process designed to identify those people who:

- you would like to get to know;
- you register initially as having something in common with;
- you would rather like to avoid.

You may prefer doing business with clients you like, but can you afford to make this distinction and run the risk of losing valued custom? Besides, you may have to suspend judgement on the client until you know more about them.

In business you cannot be so selective. It is the client who has that prerogative since they are the buyer and you are the seller. If you transmit signals that are not favourably received, you are likely to create a negative impression. It is therefore of utmost importance that you learn how to gauge and balance your presentational style between seeking involvement with your client and establishing your individuality.

# A balanced performance

Cheating in your presentation of self and style by pretending to be someone you are not is something you may do from time to time to impress others. You might create a fictional character, a person you might like to be or at least who you would like people to think you are. However, it is likely that it will backfire, especially as it becomes difficult to keep the pretence of the charade going for a long time. Although looks and appearance do matter, they will never compensate for a lack of ability. The image you project is only effective if it is accepted by others. You can fool somebody part of the time but not all the time, and are likely only to win their disapproval and create a negative impression.

Some people make more convincing actors, and the props and social graces will certainly help to create the illusion. However, the Oscar-winning role will depend on your:

- Being able to 'read' and understand the script (see Part II, The Relationship);
- Maintaining the delicate balancing act between seeking involvement with your clients and expressing your individuality;
- Mood.

Your ability to present yourself successfully and to interact well with your clients will depend on maintaining this balancing act. You must be prepared to aim for a state of involvement, where there is a higher degree of collaboration on your part enabling you to appeal to clients' emotional needs, as well as to meet your goals and to fit in with your mood and your specific role.

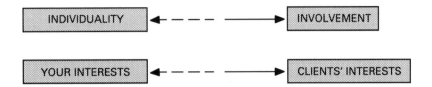

Thus do you wish to seek *involvement* by making every effort to:

- Be identified with different client groups?
- Seek clients' approval?
- Be sensitive to their needs?
- Be accepted by clients?
- Copy others?
- Conform to peer pressures? } For staff-to-staff interaction
- Uphold salon policies?

Or do you wish to exert your *individuality* by

- Drawing attention to your achievements?
- Signalling your ideologies?
- Openly expressing yourself?
- Looking after your own interests?
- Being assertive?
- Wishing to dominate?
- Drawing attention to your status?
- Rebelling?

You need to be something of a chameleon, able to adapt to the environment in which you find yourself. You must therefore be aware of your surroundings, which provide the backdrop to your performance. Hence you will need:

- To conform to certain rules, regulations and standards;
- At times to stand out, and at other times to fit in;
- To be able to adapt your presentational style to cater for different client types;
- During the course of your career to adapt to a different place of work;
- To adapt quickly to other work situations.

In all instances you must be in harmony, and need to style your presentation to make it appropriate to the script.

# Your style behaviour

The image you project to your clients is only effective if they accept it. If you send out mixed or wrong signals, you will have nobody to blame but yourself if they are misread. It will leave you feeling frustrated about yourself, and the client will be left only with negative impressions and doubt about you.

If you want to make improvements, the hardest thing is to be objective about how you present yourself. First ask yourself the following questions:

☐ What type of clients do you attract?

☐ What type of person do you attract socially?

☐ How well do you think you project yourself?

☐ Do you inspire confidence and trust?

☐ Do clients feel at ease in your company?

☐ Is there any part of your personal presentation that is letting you down?

The best people to answer these and give you positive feedback will be your clients. Put yourself in their role. Would they perceive you as:

- Being a dedicated follower of fashion trying too hard to establish an identity which is not you?
- Being a stereotype of a role model, or friend, or a slave to the media or a particular subculture in society in an attempt to stand out?
- Being a style rebel, dressing to shock?
- Having poor interpersonal skills, which may reflect your desire to assert your individuality?
- Being inconsistent in how you look, talk and act?
- Presenting an out-of-date image?
- Being a clone, where 'an image' has been made for you?

## Examples

- If you work in a salon that caters for a young, trendy clientele, you may be seen as out of place wearing a conservative-looking outfit, an unfashionable hairstyle and no make-up, and asking for the music to be turned down.
- If you are a newly established stylist working in a salon that attracts an

older clientele, they might feel intimidated if you dressed in your club gear, talked rapidly, dropped your aitches and chewed gum.

■ If you are a more senior stylist working in a fashionable salon, wearing clothes that you wore five years ago, your look may be out of date. Have you considered reassessing your wardrobe?

■ If you are a manager of a salon, you may need to dress the part. As a director of a company once said, 'All managers need to wear a jacket to look as though they are in authority'. This may seem conservative but in the professional business world there are unwritten rules on the code of dress that is considered acceptable. This does not mean looking dull, boring or unstylish. It is up to you to interpret the guidelines in a creative way.

■ If you turn up for working looking as if you have just fallen out of bed, your hair unkempt, your make-up not done, and your shoes dirty, then you deserve to be sent home to tidy yourself up.

■ If you turn up for work shirt unbuttoned to your navel and wearing a pair of faded jeans, then you may be considered inappropriately dressed to receive clients.

■ Likewise, turning up for an interview wearing an off-the-shoulder number with a plunging neckline, the interviewer might be more interested in your physical assets than in your work assets.

■ If you are immaculately styled and groomed but as soon as you speak you let yourself down by the way you talk, it may be time to change and improve your verbal skills.

A successful encounter is about interaction. It will depend on adapting your style behaviour to comply with the rules. If you are unhappy with this, you may have to clarify your role and goals.

# Adapting

You can probably reflect back to some occasion or situation and remember how self-conscious you may have been about your appearance or some other aspect of your presentation. Perhaps you didn't feel comfortable in the company of others, or perhaps you didn't have anything in common and hence felt out of place. From the way the company reacted to you, you didn't feel accepted. Consequently, you didn't present yourself well.

You are more likely to feel poised if you are dressed appropriately and are confident with your social skills. If you do not feel confident, your feelings will show, especially as our body language can be a complete give-away.

Consider the following situations and occasions:

*Work*

- Salon work
- Business meeting
- Presentation
- Training session
- TV interview
- Job interview

*Social*

- Lunch appointment
- A date
- Wedding ceremony
- Clubbing it
- Dinner party

Each has its own set of rules. All it may take is a fine tuning of your total image to give you that element of style.

Adapting means creating the correct impressions. Before deciding on what statement you want to make through the different elements of style, your performance and success at work can be greatly enhanced by evaluating:

- your needs: what you hope to achieve;
- your position, role and responsibilities;
- your place of work and other work locations;
- special functions and occasions related to work.

It was Alison Lurie who suggested that if you wear the clothing which other people think is appropriate to a situation, it signals that you are actively involved; wearing clothing that is thought 'inappropriate' sets you apart from what is taking place and others tend to exclude you.

Your total image must enable you:

- to show respect
- to get respect
- to be considerate
- not to intimidate
- to be inviting
- to show warmth and friendliness
- to set an example

- to reassure others
- to instil confidence and trust in your dependability
- to look successful
- to attract
- to look effective
- to look the part
- convey status

# 8
# The Elements of Style

## Introduction

You cannot prevent the signals representing your total image from being read by others, but what you can prevent is others judging you unfairly. To do this you must:

- ☐ Allow your personality, the true you, to shine.

- ☐ Assess and develop your clothing image.

- ☐ Understand the power of colour harmony and colour coordination.

- ☐ Work on developing your hair image.

- ☐ Improve your make-up skills.

- ☐ Not underestimate the importance of good grooming.

- ☐ Develop your awareness of non-verbal communication (body language).

- ☐ Polish your talking and listening (communication) skills.

- ☐ Improve the non-verbal characteristics of your vocal image.

## An appearance appetizer

It has been said that if you were to walk around without any clothes on your body type would reflect particular personality traits. On this principle, body shapes have been divided by some into the following types:

- Slender-boned bodies or *ectomorphs*, who are said to be introverted, sensitive and highly strung.

- The fuller figure or *endomorphs*, who are perceived as being warm, kind, jolly and reliable.
- Muscular bodies or *mesomorphs*, who are said to be independent, outgoing and well balanced.

These terms are still used today. However, since the wearing of clothes is the norm, we need to consider the signals our clothes give to others. As I already noted, personality types can be described in terms of degrees of extroversion and introversion, which give rise to a number of 'style personalities' and a clothing image.

## Clothing image

Clothes are an ingredient of style, and serve to provide protection, to preserve our modesty, to convey our status and to create an impression.

Clothes can be used to enhance one's body language. What better way to add strength to your ideologies, increase your power of getting attention or assert your domination? People who recognize the power of dress and wear clothes associated with high status tend to have much more influence than those wearing clothes associated with lower status.

First impressions give vital clues in our society that convey to others our inner emotions, intentions, lifestyle, warmth, confidence and personality. How do we read these clothing signals? What clues give the game away?

The clues are to be found within the distinguishing characteristics of each article of clothing:

- the way it is designed
- the fabric it is made from
- its colour.

A more structured style of garment is more appropriate for work that is more formal. Both the cut and choice of fabric play an important role in giving the outfit a structured shape. Work of a more informal nature such as on the shop floor might warrant a less structured approach, calling for a garment that is less formally cut and is in a much looser fabric.

Since our body shapes are unique to us and are made up of various combinations of body lines, it is important that when it comes to choosing a garment you consider how best you can flatter your figure. Aim to create visual balance to suit your proportions. It is the cut of the garment which controls the shape of the fabric or how it hangs on your body and therefore how well figure faults can be disguised. The exterior shape of a garment is known as its silhouette.

The interior shape of a garment can be achieved by incorporating style lines into the overall design. Style lines may be created by necklines, collars, lapels, waistlines, sleeves, hemlines, pockets, buttons and other design decorations, and can be used to make an outfit look more special, to add to its overall impact and to help to create proportion. The four basic style lines are curved, horizontal, diagonal and vertical. Curved lines can give a softer appeal to a garment, whilst sharp lines look harder. Since we all perceive and respond to shapes differently, you can work with different style lines to create different impressions and convey appropriateness. A softly contrasted suit can give the impression of being more relaxed, warmer and accessible, compared with a formally constructed suit which can suggest the need to dominate, be in control or exert authority. Too much glitz on a garment may be inappropriate for the world of business, may be seen as too flashy and may distract an observer from hearing you properly. Besides, it is likely to date very quickly.

The overall look of a garment will be heavily influenced by your choice of fabric. Texture, weight, lustre, print size and drapability need to be considered carefully to ensure that:

- They are compatible for your figure.
- The fabric moves or drapes well.
- The fabric is practical for the time of year.
- It is practical for work.
- It can be cleaned easily.
- It is comfortable to wear, neither too hot nor too cold.
- The fabric is suitable for different occasions.
- It conveys the right impression about you to the observer.

Naturally, how much you are prepared to spend will be determined by your budget and the image you want to create, although money is no passport to instant style appeal. When it comes to planning the perfect wardrobe, think colour, quality and classic, in that order.

## Colour

No aspect of your style is as important and emotive as colour. Subject to fashion trends, few would deny that they have colour preferences. These preferences may well be related to the degree of extroversion and introversion in your personality.

Used carefully, colour can be a powerful means of conveying the right impression and of boosting your self-confidence. Used wrongly it can diminish your appeal. The wrong colours can play amazing tricks on your skin tones, making you look tired, haggard and older and giving you a pasty complexion. More flattering colours will enhance your natural colouring, accentuate your eyes, and make your skin look clear and healthy.

The speed factor is guaranteed to get you noticed. The eye registers colours at different speeds as follows:

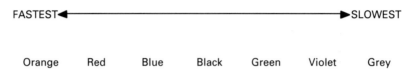

FASTEST◀——————————————————————————————▶SLOWEST

Orange    Red    Blue    Black    Green    Violet    Grey

Getting yourself noticed may be one good reason for wearing high energy colours. For many, however, colour is a signal of ambition, so darker neutrals such as greys, navies, browns and black are firm business favourites. Those who dislike forward planning and like taking risks will tend to prefer the brighter colours, especially greens, reds, light blues and orange.

The world of colour emotions and associations makes for interesting study. Much research has been conducted on the psychology of colour and its effect on the wearer and the observer, and on whether it reflects how one is feeling. We draw upon colour traits daily in the hope that we can learn more about the people we meet. However, it is important to bear in mind that some colours convey mixed messages.

Have you ever tried on a number of outfits one after the other, say before going to work or out socially, only to be unhappy with your final choice? When this happens, it may also be due to the design. However, the real problem may well be the colour, especially if it has not got the same vibrational energy as you that day. If the colour is not right for you that day, you will not be happy. The colour you choose should represent the inner you. It needs to reflect how you feel that day, that is, your mood.

On those occasions when you are dressing and you look at yourself in the mirror, have you ever asked yourself the question, 'What does this colour do for me?' Think about this now.

- Do you look best in light, medium or dark colours?
- Do warmer colours suit you better than cooler ones?
- Can you wear colours that are neither warm nor cool?
- Do you look better in brighter, softer or muted colours?

In order to look your best, you need to appreciate which colours flatter your overall colour profile, taking into consideration your hair, eye and skin tones and dominant colour characteristics.

The first step is to assess what colour your skin tone is. Made up of varying amounts of colour pigments, your complexion is based on either yellow or blue. It is these undertones in your skin which affect how you look in different colours. If your complexion is yellow based your skin has a warm undertone, and if it is blue based it has a cool undertone. Skin is said to be of medium undertone if it has both warm and cool characteristics. Those who have such a skin tone will suit a range of warm and cool colours.

The intensity of your overall colouring, how light or dark you appear, will influence how strong a colour you can suitably wear.

To achieve the right amount of colour contrast in what you wear, observe the contrast between your hair and skin tones. This contrast influences the clarity of your colours, how bright, soft or muted they need to be.

Learning how colours are derived, and working out your colour profile and the colours that are most flattering to you and how you can wear them, are central to the technique of colour analysis. Much has been said about the rigidity of the technique and the cloning effect of certain systems over the years. This is the fault not so much of the technique as of how a client is initially assessed and the way in which the results are interpreted and the recommendations are made and then acted upon. Used with awareness, a tonal approach to colour can be both an art and a science. It can be used to greatly enhance your appearance, as well as to bring an exciting new dimension to hair colouring and make-up services (see Appendix 2).

## Quality

The argument for buying a quality article of clothing or accessory is based on

- its exclusivity;
- more attention having been paid to its construction (e.g. seams, stitching, buttons and collars);
- better manufacture, using the skills of the designer and cutter;
- the use of more expensive fabric;
- better fit;
- better quality control in its production.

These are all good reasons why paying that little bit extra for something often means that it is going to be working for you longer (have a longer hanger life), particularly if it is of classic design.

Classics are those timeless, simple, well cut clothes that avoid high fashion gimmicks and provide endless versatile options for dressing for different occasions, especially with the help of up-to-date accessories.

## Accessories

Accessories can often make or break your total look. Used cleverly, they can transform the mood of your clothes from day into night or give that good old faithful classic black dress extra oomph. They can be used as a focal point to attract attention, and can alter the visual balance of your body proportions.

There is much to be said for buying and building up a collection of good quality accessories such as costume jewellery, a decent watch, classic leather belts to suit your figure, comfortable shoes and practical bags.

## Grooming

Since we are in a grooming business where impressions are easily made, no amount of fashion styling will substitute for poor grooming. Grooming is the very foundation of looking great and improving your attractiveness. It says:

- you care
- you spend time on yourself
- you take the trouble
- you respect yourself.

A slatternly, unkempt or scruffy appearance may imply

- a lack of self-worth
- laziness
- a lack of foresight, causing you to leave insufficient time
- a lack of respect for others.

If your hair doesn't look good, if your skin care, body care and make-up are poor, they will detract from your total look and convey only negative impressions about you. They may be only very small details, but must never be overlooked.

In this age, when we all have complex lifestyles, time is of the essence. If it means getting up that bit earlier before work to attend to your personal appearance, then do so. Late nights are no excuse for untidiness. Effective time management is an important factor in maintaining a consistently high standard. Planning and good routine will allow you to book time with yourself and get you into the routine of practising good habits.

As children we were encouraged to take care of ourselves and perform daily personal activities. Many are habits that should be second nature; others are good practices that need to be adopted. Don't expect your clients or customers to tell you directly, so please excuse me if I mention them.

## Body care

- Have a daily shower or bath to eliminate body odour.
- Use an underarm deodorant.
- Choose your perfume or after-shave carefully.
- Use waxing or other forms of hair removal.

## Face care

- Daily skin-care programme for both men and women to promote healthy-looking skin.
- Well shaven faces for men.
- Well applied make-up for women.
- Flattering jewellery to enhance the shape of your face.

## Hair care

- It should go without saying that a hairdresser must have clean, healthy, well cut and well styled hair.

## Dental care

- Regular dental check-ups and visits to the dental hygienist are essential for healthy teeth and gums. So too is regular brushing, morning, noon and night. Bad breath is offensive; so too is garlic, alcohol and cigarette smoke. If necessary use a breath-freshener spray or a mouthwash.
- If you are unhappy with the way your teeth look, you may be unable to smile with confidence. You should therefore seek professional advice about how to improve your teeth. It's money well spent.

## Eye care

- If you need to wear glasses and are self-conscious about this, get professional advice on what style of frames would best suit your face shape or seek out a reputable contact lens practitioner. There's no point having impaired vision or damaging your eyes through your vanity.

## Hand care

- Since we use our hands so much and they are always in focus, ensure that nails are clean and well manicured. Long dirty finger nails are a complete turn-off. So too are badly painted, chipped nails or nails that have been bitten.

## Foot care

- Standing all day is a strain on the body. It is therefore important that you take care of your feet by wearing suitable footwear. If necessary, book a session with the chiropodist to sort out any foot troubles or for routine foot care.

## Well-being

- Prevention is better than cure. Most health practices offer routine medical check-ups and screening for both men and women. Don't ignore the importance of good diet, exercise, rest and stress control.

## Clothes care

- It is natural for the body to perspire, so it is essential to wear once and then wash any garment that is worn next to the skin to avoid the build-up of body odour in the fabric.
- Clothes that cannot be washed should be dry cleaned regularly.
- Brush your clothes down to remove hair and dust, etc.
- Hang your clothes on quality hangers to help them keep their shape.
- Avoid buying clothes that are too light.
- Repair missing buttons, loose hems or hanging threads.
- Clothes that have creases or knife-like pleats should be pressed regularly.
- Avoid wearing clothes that are too tight.
- Coordinate the colour of your hosiery with your hemline or shoe colour.

- Hosiery with holes in is unimpressive.

## Shoe care

- Daily cleansing of leather or brushing of suede is essential to remove dirt and scruff marks.
- Replace broken laces.
- Have shoes soled and heeled when necessary. Badly worn-down shoes are unimpressive.
- Keep your shoes in good shape with shoe trees, and protect them with a recommended protector.

# Developing your appearance

- Allow your personality, the true you, to shine.
- Put your stamp of individuality on what you wear and how you wear it.
- Whatever you wear, put it on with confidence and wear it with confidence.
- Lean to love your body and like yourself. Play on your assets and strengths. We all have good points, regardless of our height and weight.
- Let your clothes enhance the positive and minimize the not so positive parts of your body.
- Create a totally balanced body without treating a particular feature in isolation.
- Don't ignore the importance of good posture.
- Your clothes should be appropriate for your position at work as well as your social activities.
- Ensure that your clothes fit well, and buy the best that you can afford.
- Enhance your facial image by ensuring that the colours of clothes that sit closest to your face are the most flattering for your colouring.
- Learn how to mix and match colours that suit you. Appreciate the power of colour. Do people notice you first or the colours you are wearing?
- Enhance your facial image by choosing a haircut or style to suit your face shape and features.
- Plan a routine beauty and hair-maintenance programme.
- Add an extra dimension to your face by wearing correctly colour-balanced make-up.
- Use make-up to camouflage any facial imperfections.

- Create extra facial interest by wearing eye-catching accessories such as glasses or ear-rings.
- Ensure that all facial accessories suit your face shape and features.
- Enhance your body shape by wearing clothes and accessories to suit your figure image.
- Learn how to use accessories as focal points.
- Keep an open mind about fashion.
- Adapt fashion to suit your needs.
- Spend time at first window shopping.
- Remember that practice makes perfect.
- Have fun and enjoy looking your best.

# Communication skills

Communicating is something we do every day of our lives. We all know how to communicate in one form or another, perhaps without even thinking about it. You will need to be an effective communicator at all levels, whether talking to a client face to face, addressing a group of people or giving a seminar.

In this section I will be looking at person-to-person communication. Put simply, communication is the exchange of information. When you speak to a client, your voice tone and pitch, your selection of words, your facial expression and your eye contact all convey information about you. Of the first impression, fifty-five per cent is based on your appearance and body language, and thirty-eight per cent is based on how you speak: your vocal image. The words you use account for seven per cent. The client interprets all of these and judges you in the light of their own attitudes and beliefs.

I'm sure that during the course of your work you meet a wide cross-section of people. At times you may have a client who is more challenging, not necessarily technically or artistically. Perhaps they have a more complex personality, and you need to have your wits about you and to draw upon a range of communication skills to win that client over. These skills require you to:

Develop an understanding of body language. This will equip you with the ability not only to read clients' subconscious messages better but also to make sure that you are sending out appropriate body signals and can make them work for you.

Develop your talking and listening skills. Ask many people what they consider to be the most important aspect of communicating and they will probably say 'talking'. However, we also need to consider the importance of listening. Nothing is more infuriating to someone than the impression that everything they have said has 'gone in one ear and out of the other'.

Without two-way communication you are alone; you have no means of:

- registering your feelings
- understanding a client's needs
- gathering information about them
- making assessments and evaluations
- sharing your ideas
- showing you are really interested and care.

If there is no effective communication between you and your client, there is no interaction and little chance of establishing a relationship.


# Body language

In this technological age we have developed complex systems that permit us to transmit and receive signals around the world in a matter of minutes, enabling us to communicate messages with ease, efficiency and accuracy.

No less complex is the way we communicate with one another, face to face. The messages we give through our appearance are only one important aspect of our interaction, and, together with our network of non-verbal signals or clues called body language, we have a system that can be used to aid our communication process. Before you even speak, these silent communicators are already broadcasting messages to the people you meet. If you are saying one thing and your body language says something totally different, don't be surprised if you are treated with caution and fail to impress.

For any person in a business that relies on precise interaction, good body language skills are an essential element of style, not only for projecting yourself but also to enable you to read the emotions of others. Star performers know how to integrate appropriate clues of the right intensity to suit their audience. They ensure that the different channels of communication work in harmony with one another. These channels comprise:

- Eye contact
- Facial expression
- Head movements
- Gestures and body movements
- Posture and body orientation
- The use of distance and space
- Body contact through touch
- Non-verbal characteristics of vocal communication
- Appearance.

These clues play an important part in our interpersonal relationships and serve as signals at the various stages of an encounter. There are three kinds of clue, namely:

**Immediacy clues:** These are used to communicate either our like or dislike for another person, by how much eye contact we sustain, the extent to which we touch someone, and how far or how close we position ourselves in relation to them.

**Relaxation clues:** These come from how we position our arms and legs, our posture and how relaxed our hands and neck are. A position of asymmetry signals a more relaxed state.

**Activity clues:** These signal how responsive we feel towards another person, and are expressed by our facial mannerisms, rate of speech, gesticulation, and foot and body movements such as rocking and swivelling.

The skill lies in learning to adjust each type of clue so as to propel your client encounters successfully and smoothly from beginning to end in order to produce positive results.

## Essential body language skills

### Making eye contact

Of all the communication channels our eyes are the next most powerful means of communication after words. They are our windows to the world around us, and mirror our innermost feelings. Eyes are not only receivers of information but also transmitters of signals that play a vital role in our interaction with others.

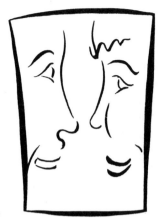

Eye contact.

From the quick fleeting look to frequent glances, from mutual gaze to a hostile stare, we use eye contact to:

■ Seek additional information from others.
■ Show attention and interest. This is often accompanied with a gesture of greeting – the 'eyebrows flash'. It is a signal that we are pleased to greet someone; a sign of recognition.
■ Show intense emotion and invite interaction.
■ Dominate, influence or threaten others, characterized by long unflickering looks.
■ Signal our intention to speak, by making eye contact with other listeners.
■ Emphasize a point whilst speaking.
■ Enhance our listening skills during conversation in order to provide positive feedback.
■ Convey our attitude and inner emotions, such as aggression, excitement, anger, fear and sadness, which all have different eye behaviours.

## Positive eye contact

Use eye contact to produce positive responses from your clients.

■ Speak to them face to face rather than into the mirror. Look at them when they are talking to you.
■ Look at them with fairly long glances. Know how to vary the amount of eye contact by introducing look-aways so they feel comfortable.

Effective communication between two persons requires each party to be happy with the amount of eye contact.

- Look more when listening to your clients and less whilst talking.
- Look away when taking up the conversation from your clients. Look back when giving them the floor.
- Use positive facial expressions such as smiling combined with eye contact to convey warmth and friendliness.
- Let your eyes show excitement, keenness and happiness.

## Negative eye contact

The following eye behaviours are certain to create a negative impression with your clients:

Too little eye contact can be seen as being a sign of:

- lack of interest
- impoliteness
- insincerity
- shyness
- nervousness
- lack of confidence
- untrustworthiness.

Too much eye contact can signal:

- a feeling of superiority
- a lack of respect
- hostility and anger
- over-familiarity and physical attraction.

Your emotions can say

- anger (eyes narrow)
- sadness (looking down)
- fear (eyes become 'frozen').

## Facial expressions

Faces fascinate us. They can attract, offend, repel or even frighten. The Ancient Greeks studied the art of physiognomy. They believed that by studying face shapes and expressions they could predict personality types. We can learn a great deal about a person's emotional state by observing their face. In terms of body language, facial expressions are second only to eye signals as the most powerful means of expressing our emotions.

If you watch a play or television programme, you will see that the actors often take their cues from the expressions of fellow actors. When you are talking to clients, concentrate on what they are saying. Look at their face for expressions and emotions which will give you additional information and also tell you when it is the right moment to respond.

Be aware of your own expression. It can encourage your client to continue enthusiastically and to enjoy talking to you.

## Types of facial expression

American researchers Paul Eckman and Wallace Friesan discovered that the emotions we experience can be grouped certain four basic types (see Part II, The Relationship), each producing a different facial expression.

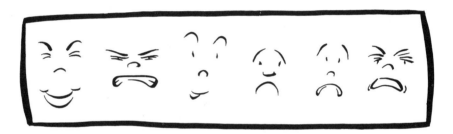

Facial expressions: happy, angry, interested, sad, scared, disgusted.

- **Happiness.** This can range from a slight to normal to broad smile or grin, depending on the position of the mouth, cheeks and how much the teeth are shown.

- **Anger.** This is characterized by a lengthy gaze, frowning or scowling and a gritting of the teeth together. It is not uncommon for facial and body muscles to tense up when a person is angry and for skin tone to redden.

- **Interest.** A person can be seen to cock their head at an angle towards another person if they are interested in what they are saying. At the same time the eyes appear larger than normal and the person may have an open mouth.

- **Sadness.** A feeling of sadness will be displayed by a general lack of expression, little eye contact and a down turned mouth.

☐ **Fear.** This is evident from wide open eyes, an open mouth, trembling or paleness of colour and even perspiration.

☐ **Disgust.** It shows itself in a wrinkled nose and raised upper lip. The lower eyelid is pushed up and the brows are lowered.

## Positive facial expressions

■ Use the power of the smile to get off to a good start. The smile is a great greeting, signalling to your clients that you are pleased to see them. It can also convey pleasure and happiness.
■ Vary your facial expression to move the client towards a happy state.
■ Use facial expressions such as the 'head cock' to show you are a good listener.
■ Animate your speaking by using appropriate facial expressions to make your conversation more interesting.

## Negative facial impressions

■ Staring at a blank wall is uninteresting. So too is talking to a blank face. This may give the impression of lack of interest or even hostility.
■ Badly contrived expressions may give the impression that you are insincere.
■ Closing your eyes is enough to say 'I'm not interested.'
■ Frowning.

## Using your head

If two people are observed in conversation, it will be seen that, as well as varying their eye contact and facial expression, they will move their heads in different ways depending on whether they are talking or listening. Adapting these skills you can use a variety of head movements to help you communicate more effectively with clients.

Head movements can be used during talking to:

■ express your attitude to your client;
■ add emphasis to how you speak and what you say;
■ act as a baton to direct the flow of conversation.

They can be used when listening to:

■ enable you to focus directly on your clients when they are speaking;

■ show that you agree with, approve and accept what they are saying.

The most common head movements are the

■ **Head nod:** A rhythmic up-and-down action of the head. Continued movement during conversation is a sign of attention and interest.
■ **Head cock:** Here your head is tilted at an angle to the client and can be used to say, 'I'm interested in what you are saying'.

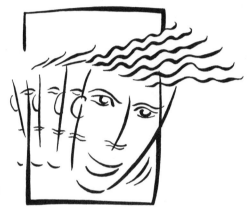

Positive head movements:
head cock.

## Positive head movements

■ Use the head nod as a means of acknowledgement during the first encounter: as a gesture of greeting.
■ If you wish to express doubt, the head can be gently rocked from side to side.
■ To say 'No' the head can be shaken.
■ To say to somebody in a playful way 'Let's keep it a secret between the two of us', use the wink.
■ Vary the strength of the nod from single to double nods to signal feedback when the client is talking to show how well you understand and agree with what they are saying.
■ Use the head nod to encourage your clients to speak more freely.
■ To add emphasis to your words, nod the head using small downward movements.

## Negative head movements

■ Holding your head high and tilting it backwards conveys an air of superiority.

- Lowering your head suggests you are submissive. It can also indicate a low self-esteem.
- Using your head to beckon the client to follow you is impolite.
- Tossing your head backwards expresses disdain.

## Let your body talk

Gestures and body movements are another useful channel of non-verbal communication. I'm sure you have at times played the game 'charades' where you have to communicate to other players a selected title phrase without using words. If, through your actions and movements, they are able to guess the title, you have given a successful performance.

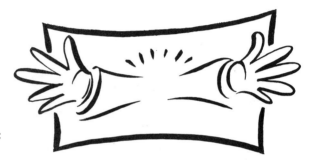

Body language:
hand gestures.

In the salon we are not limited to silent actions. Nevertheless we can use gestures to add interest and animation to 'colour' our interaction and conversation with clients. I have already discussed the use of the head in making gestures. I will now focus on the action of our arms, hands and fingers to:

- express your personality
- express a point
- express your attitude.

Imagine you are a conductor of an orchestra, using your hands to control the tempo and to introduce different sections of the orchestra and fade out others. In much the same way, you can use your hands to 'talk' to your clients and punctuate what you say. How delicately you use your hands will enhance the client's perception of your artistic qualities and convey an impression of precision in your work. If you want to give the impression of drive and determination, speed up the hand signals, but don't overdo them.

## Positive hand and arm actions

- Use the open palm as a gesture of openness towards your client.
- A downward baton-like action of the hand can be used to add emphasis to what you say.
- The 'precision grip' combines a crab-like movement of the thumb and forefinger to emphasize a delicate point.
- 'Thumbs-up' conveys to the client 'your hair looks good'.
- A sweep of the lower arm from the elbow in a certain direction away from your body says 'After you' or 'Kindly go first'.
- When the fingertips of each hand are placed together and the palms are kept apart it signals confidence to a listener.
- You can use your hands to 'talk' shape, movement, length and other style characteristics.

## Negative hand and arm actions

- Wringing your hands whilst standing talking to a client says you are anxious.
- Pointing can convey hostility.
- Clenching your fist can signal that you are over-determined to the point of being aggressive.
- Standing with your hands on your hips is a sign that you want to assert yourself.
- Standing with your arms folded forms a barrier between you and your client.
- Avoid hands in the pockets. It may be seen as a desire to dominate.
- Crossing your fingers whilst talking to a client is a gesture of protection and may indicate that you are not very confident.
- Standing behind a client and, whilst talking to them, preening oneself in the mirror is not only extremely bad manners, but also a signal of invitation saying, 'Look at me'!
- Excessive gesturing when a client is talking may make you appear over-keen to speak.
- Touching your face whilst talking may indicate that you are anxious.

Just as your gestures will give vital clues about your personality and attitude, it is important to be aware of the gesture responses and body movements made by your clients. These can offer clues to how the client may feel about the experience (see Chapter 9, The Consultation).

To summarize, open and positive gestures and actions will be more favourably received by your clients as a genuine attempt to communicate warmth, trust and friendship. Actions often speak louder than words.

## Posture

For well over a hundred years interest has been growing among alternative medical and fitness practitioners in the relationship between the mind and the body and how we use it. One such form of body awareness was developed by F. Matthias Alexander (1869–1955). The Alexander Technique teaches awareness of posture and movement and how to maintain balance and poise with minimal tension. Less stress is what we all need if we are to perform at our peak.

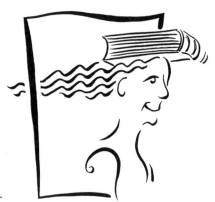

Body language: positive posturing.

As children our first introduction to 'appearance training' was being told to stand up straight in preference to slouching. Girls at finishing schools are disciplined in the traditional art of walking with books balanced on their heads to help them improve their deportment and 'walk tall', as well as how to sit elegantly and get in and out of cars in a ladylike fashion. Models learn how to stand and walk to best display fashion garments.

These skills and techniques are extremely valuable in everyday life to improve our health, fitness and appearance, but we should not overlook the valuable contribution posture makes to body language. Posture is an expression of ourselves, our personality, moods, self-image and attitude to others.

In this section we will look at how to generate warmth and friendliness and make your clients more willing to interact with you.

## Positive posture

- To look elegantly taller, keep your shoulders back and your stomach in. Avoid becoming too round shouldered, developing a stoop or allowing your head to sag. Practise posture exercises as well as learning how to use your legs to support your body.
- When standing talking to a client, adopt a fairly erect open posture, with your arms held loosely down by the sides of your body. The more erect your posture, the more confident you will appear. Open posture signals that you are interested and willing to help.
- If you want to appear relaxed, lean sideways slightly but take care not to appear too casual.
- Turn your entire body in the direction of the client.
- Leaning forwards in a relaxed manner is a way of convincing clients you like them.

## Negative posture

- Standing with your hands on your hips is a sign of a desire to dominate.
- Forming a body barrier by folding your arms across your chest is a sign of unwillingness to listen or of a lack of interest in your client.
- Standing erect with your head back indicates you are trying to put across high status.
- Conversely, lower status is often displayed by the bowing of the head and by submissive body positions, such as the hands held behind the back. If this is overdone, you will not generate confidence.
- Standing with your hands by your side with your fists clenched is a sign of aggression.
- Standing and talking with your head bowed can say you are shy, submissive and less than confident.
- Using the shoulder shrug while standing, accompanied by negative facial expressions and head movements and having the arms raised with palms upwards, says that you don't know or care.
- If a man stands with thumbs hooked over the belt or into the trouser pockets, with the fist loosely clenched, it's a sign of sexual invitation.

In our posture discussion so far, the client is sitting down and you are talking to them standing up. You may find a client responds better if you sit down and speak to them on their level, making eye-to-eye contact instead of looking down on them. This is a masterly piece of body orientation, designed to make interaction easier and more relaxed. For this you must make sure that you position a stool next to your client's chair.

### Positive sitting postures

- When your client is talking, adopt a more open posture, leaning your head and trunk to one side and leaving your legs and arms uncrossed. This is a posture of agreement.
- As your interest develops, lean forward towards your client, with your legs drawn back.

### Negative sitting postures

- There are closed postures where the head and trunk are held straight and the arms and legs are crossed. These signal a very defensive state and are habits that are likely to be very hard to break.
- A crossed arm and hand to the face says you are sceptical of what is being said.
- Boredom or complete lack of interest is evident from outstretched body leaning backwards with legs stretched out.

## Body contact

As babies touch was vital in our early development. We looked to our parents, particularly our mother, for tactile pleasures that would give us comfort and reassurance. Touch gave us an early means of communicating with others, which we have carried through into adult life.

Although as adults we have become more inhibited about touch, most probably due to social rules of acceptability, we nevertheless know what the power of touch can do in certain situations. It can be used to show support, give encouragement, offer sympathy, and express appreciation, affection and attraction. In a tactile profession such as hairdressing, we become confident about using our hands in a functional way which carries no message. It is accepted that we can touch even the head, neck and shoulders, vulnerable areas of the body that are normally out of bounds except in intimate relationships. Only the arm offers a non-vulnerable area of safe body contact. This trust to touch is shared with only a few professions and does not carry a licence for wandering hands!

Besides touch having a functional use, we use it as a means of greeting as in the handshake, the kiss on first meeting or on parting, or when listening to a client to offer reassurance. As with other forms of body language we need to recognize how we use it. We need to be aware of who we are touching, where we touch, how we touch, how long the touch lasts, and when the time is right, if we are not to make a client feel uncomfortable.

It is essential to develop the use of touch along with other body language skills so that it does not appear to be out of context.

### Positive body contact

- Use a fairly positive handshake as a gesture of greeting and parting. However, be aware that this carries messages. In men a limp-wristed handshake is thought to be effeminate or to indicate a weaker personality type. In women a weak handshake may be taken as showing a reluctance to interact or insincerity.
- Kissing on the cheeks as a gesture of greeting and parting should be reserved for those clients whom you know very well and with whom you have developed a special relationship over a period of time.
- If, when you are talking to a client, they seem uneasy about your advice, use a reassuring touch on their forearm or shoulder.
- If, during conversation with a client, you can see that they need your emotional support, use a gentle holding touch on their arm.

I will return to Body Language in Part IV but now let us consider developing your vocal image.

## Vocal image

Have you ever been in the presence of somebody who holds you spellbound by the way they speak? On how many occasions have you met somebody and been impressed by their appearance, only to be let down by the way they talk?

Our voices not only help to paint vivid pictures that affect how people see us, but also indicate how we see ourselves. What does your voice tell people about you? Does your voice enhance your overall total image?

The voice is an important part of your overall total image and if used effectively can capture your clients' full attention, especially if:

- They can easily understand you.
- You are pleasant to listen to.
- You are expressive in what you say.

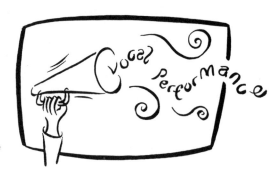

Does your voice enhance
your total image?

## How to use your vocal image to influence others

### *Projection*

☐ Whether you are talking to a client or an audience, make sure you can be heard. It makes you stand out and seem as if you are bubbling over with confidence.

☐ Clear, precise speech allows you to put definition between your words. It also gives your mind a chance to catch up with your words, and it allows you to put facial expressions in where needed. More than anything it will make it easier for your clients to understand you.

☐ If you need to add more impact and interest, use pauses and variations in loudness to emphasize words or phrases.

☐ Use your natural pitch and normal breathing pattern to produce the best quality sound with minimum effort.

☐ Being expressive will help you to 'colour' what you say and to share your inner emotions.

☐ Use the right tone of voice to convey the correct messages. Regardless of the words you use, your tone of voice will instantly convey to a client:

- friendliness
- warmth
- confidence
- interest
- mood
- frustration
- anger.

## Tonal quality

It's not what you say, but how you say it!'

How many times have you heard this phrase being used? By varying the tone of your voice you can decrease your clients' negative emotions and maximize their positive ones. This skill can be used to great effect to influence your client's feelings about themselves and their attitude to you.

By imitating your client's vocal tone you reinforce the quality they are trying to convey. Thus, if a client is talking slowly or fast, alter your rate of speaking accordingly. A warm friendly tone in your client's voice should be met with a similar tone.

By matching and elevating your client's tone you can heighten the quality they are conveying. In this way you can increase their confidence, give compliments and increase overall enthusiasm.

Using a tone opposite that of your client's voice brings out the quality opposite the one they are conveying. For instance, since people usually experience the emotion their voice expresses, getting your client to imitate your positive voice can effectively change their feelings. This can be useful when speaking with your clients in a variety of situations. You can increase good feelings with a tone of voice that is more intense. By choosing the right one you can:

- reduce anxiety and apprehension
- heighten reassurance
- elevate enthusiasm and awareness
- reduce aggression
- overcome moods
- pacify dissatisfaction
- soothe minor irritations
- promote warmth, sincerity and friendliness.

For this to work effectively you need to listen really carefully to your clients and observe their body language. This will enable you to deduce what their inner feelings are from how they are speaking.

Conversely, if you speak with a negative tone – if you sound intimidating, aggressive, uninterested, unsure – you will not easily win clients over.

## Vocal quality

Are you speaking unclearly, mumbling or cutting short your sentences?

☐    Is the rate at which you are speaking too fast, too slow or too constant?

☐    Is your voice pitched too high or too low?

☐    Are you speaking too loudly or too softly for the situation?

☐    Do you use pauses and variations in loudness for emphasis and to add interest?

☐    Are you introducing variations in tone in your speech?

☐    Is your speech expressive?

# PART IV
# INTERPRETING THE CLIENT'S NEEDS

# 9
# *The Consultation*

## An integrated approach

No other part of our body is as versatile as our hair. It is an essential prop, and, if one is prepared to spend time, one can train and coax this magical material into endless shapes and styles, to create different illusions of form by careful cutting, colouring, perming, styling and dressing.

However, to avoid disappointment it is important during the initial consultation to consider carefully all limitations and restrictions that may affect suitability of a particular style.

Hair is not only the most revealing but perhaps the most powerful means of expressing personality. The style, length, colour and condition can be used to make a powerful statement. A person's hair can indeed be their 'crowning glory'. They could be wearing the latest designer clothes and accessories and have fabulous flattering make-up, but if their hair does not look good they are simply not doing themselves justice.

Every person has uniquely different features, and when planning a new hair image for a client it is crucial that you appreciate the aesthetic relationship between their head, face and body. It is essential that they all interrelate and harmonize with each other.

Just think how confident a client will feel when they know how good their hair looks. Think of it as an accessory which can be adapted to enhance their features and physique as well as to project their personality and suit their lifestyle and age.

Many clients may be under the impression that there is only one hairstyle to suit them. Perhaps they are lacking self-confidence to change their hair image after many years; perhaps they need new ideas to stimulate them.

Your style recommendations should first focus on being able to interpret their needs. Start with an in-depth evaluation of the following:

- Personality profile.
- Age considerations.
- Lifestyle considerations.
- Style aesthetics*: head, face and body details.
- Design Components*: the physical characteristics of hair; the technical aspects of cutting, colouring, perming, styling and dressing.

This evaluation must be integrated into the consultation.

# 'My hairdresser...'

Wherever I am asked to give a presentation to a group of people on how they can improve their total image, when it comes to talking about hair you can be sure that this is the aspect of appearance which gives most frustration.

These are some of the comments that people often make.

'I hate going to the hairdressers, I'd sooner go to the dentist.'
'I only wanted a trim, but they always cut my hair too short.'
'I asked for a perm and left looking like a poodle.'
'I know my hair is in a bad way but why do they make me feel like I've been a naughty girl?'
'I always feel intimidated by them and eventually say, "Well, do what you think will suit me best" and then leave wishing I hadn't said that.'
'Why is it that my hairdresser never listens to what I want?'
'I take along a picture and when I produce it they get angry.'
'Within a few minutes of being seated in the salon I am whisked away to be shampooed before getting a chance to properly discuss my needs.'

These comments and many others show that there is cause for concern. I agree that it takes time to develop the client–hairdresser relationship and that clients also need to know how they can contribute to a happy partnership, but the onus is on you, the hairdresser, to take the lead, starting with developing your consultation skills. Your aim should be to get the client involved in the process.

For the moment I will assume that a client has already booked over the phone either your services or those of a staff member. Unlike most selling situations, in this instance they have already made a conscious decision to buy. From the moment they enter the salon they are a 'captive audience'.

---

*This book assumes you have a sound knowledge in these creative and technical areas.

They would not be there in the first place unless they wanted solutions. Nevertheless you will need to proceed in a structured way, fulfilling the role of the problem solver.

## Objectives

Without doubt the consultation should provide a firm foundation on the basis of which you can:

- create the right environment;
- establish friendly personal contact;
- hear the needs, views and wishes of each client;
- convey your ideas and give advice;
- promote other services which could benefit the client;
- make recommendations;
- agree on a definite course of action.

The consultation is a crucial stage yet its importance is often overlooked. It should form an appreciable part of a client's appointment, so that all subsequent practical stages in the transformation flow smoothly, resulting in another totally satisfied customer.

This is especially important when dealing with a new client or one who has been referred to you. Assume that they know very little about you or your salon services. You will need to spend time communicating this information. Some may have vague ideas of what they want; others may need more help.

How much time do you allow for this? Five minutes, ten minutes, fifteen minutes – or longer? Just because you are busy, do you try to take short cuts in order to save time, such as getting a trainee to shampoo the client's hair before speaking to them? I hope not. This is a sure recipe for disaster. Even regular clients might on this occasion wish to have a restyle.

If you are a salon owner, it is certainly worth looking at your booking system and appointment structure in order to:

- incorporate a definite consultation stage with an appointment time;
- allow extra time for this if necessary.

You may have to restructure your fees accordingly, and in the short term you may have to lose an appointment slot in order to increase the length of all appointments. In the long term you stand to gain more satisfied clients. Think of it as an investment.

There are no short cuts to a professionally conducted consultation, and there can be no excuses. A client does not want to hear apologies for being overlooked. Most clients will understand that the best system can often be upset by factors outside your control. But what they will not tolerate is being kept waiting because you or your staff are overbooked and consequently rushed. You would not be impressed if you had booked a table for dinner at a restaurant only to be given the impression that the management were in a hurry to take your order, speed you through the meal and present you with the bill before finishing, in order to accommodate another party.

This discussion on consultation skills is a follow-on from what I said earlier about the art of selling. I will be looking at how to improve and enhance your 'chairside manner' by

- elaborating on what you want to achieve during the consultation, by applying the basic selling model, AIDA;
- describing how you can practise the power of positive first impressions;
- discussing the use of effective communication skills;
- describing how you should apply your assessment and diagnostic skills and use your hair knowledge.

# Conversational strategy

Effective communication will cement that degree of trust between you and your clients. In order for them to trust you, you need to convince the clients that you trust yourself. This means you must be able to instil confidence. Confidence breeds confidence.

## Techniques to make the consultation more meaningful

### True presence

Turn your body in the direction of your client. Look at them when they are talking to you, concentrate on what they are saying, and look at their face for expression and emotion; this will give you additional information, and also tell you when it is the right moment to respond.

COMMUNICATION PATHWAY

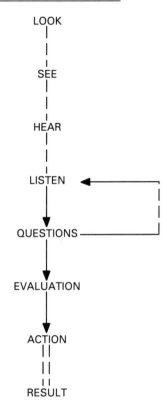

## *Open-ended questions*

Use open-ended questions to encourage your client to talk freely. This is the best way to establish their needs and problems. Remember: you are not conducting an interrogation so you need to ask the right questions and phrase them correctly, e.g. 'How', 'Why', and 'Tell me about . . .'.

## *Conversation facilitators*

Use these words or phrases to convey interest and encourage your client to continue talking about themselves:

'Tell me more.'

'That sounds interesting.'

'Do you really?'

'How about . . .?'

'Have you?'

'Tell me.'

### Reading between the lines

Make use of free information to ask appropriate questions. Free information includes not only what is said, but what you observe, e.g. first impressions such as dress, facial expression, mood, voice.

### Vary your information gathering

Use both opinions and facts, sometimes followed by a question.

### Show honesty

Be open, say what you mean, mean what you say, and share your true thoughts with your client.

### The personal touch

Use your client's name in the conversation. People like to hear their name being used.

### First person

Express your opinions, advice and feelings by using 'I consider', 'I advise', 'I feel'.

### Praise

Praising your clients about, say, their appearance or about something they have achieved helps to create a warm, friendlier environment.

## Listening

Talking certainly does play a major role in communication. However, it is vital also to consider the role of listening. I'm sure you are working or have worked in salons where music is played. In most cases it is used as background music which does not drown conversation. You hear that music is being played, although you probably hardly notice it.

Compare this with when you have been to see a well known band perform at a live concert. You may have worked your way towards the stage so that you are in the best position to hear and see the performance. The closer you get to the stage, the more you become physically influenced by the music and the lights. Your body responds, moving to the beat, you applaud, you whistle and tap to the rhythm. You are now listening.

Let us relate this to the relationship with your clients during the consultation.

## Non-judgemental listening

☐ Appreciate what is being said by your client.

☐ Be sensitive to all the words spoken.

☐ Don't dwell on trigger or emotive words that cause you to put up a block and prevent you from listening further.

☐ Do not fall into the trap of misunderstanding simply because you are not listening correctly.

☐ You may disagree, but do not let this interfere with listening fully.

## Active listening

This requires you to concentrate on what your client is feeling and/or trying to convey and to feed it back to them for confirmation or clarification.

By practising active listening you can verify your understanding of your clients' needs and get closer to their true feelings, uncover problems, eliminate alternatives and control the consultation.

Use active listening to clarify exactly what it is that your client wants. Here are some examples.

CLIENT 1: I would like a hairstyle that is easy to care for.
HAIRDRESSER: It sounds like you have a job that is very demanding.

CLIENT 2: My boyfriend does not like me with short hair.
HAIRDRESSER: What do you mean by 'short'?

CLIENT 3: I'm not very happy with the hair products I have been using.
HAIRDRESSER: Have you considered trying . . .?

# Reasons for a breakdown in communication

☐ The consultation has a disorganized structure.

☐ The right questions have not been asked.

☐ Questions have not been phrased correctly.

☐ The hairdresser has been a poor listener.

☐ The client's real needs have not been understood.

☐ There has been little eye contact.

☐ The hairdresser is not interested in the client as a person.

☐ A 'take it or leave it' attitude has been adopted.

☐ The hairdresser has been aggressive when questioning.

☐ He or she is arrogant and intimidating.

☐ He or she has no tact.

☐ There has been a lack of consideration.

☐ The hairdresser appears untrustworthy.

☐ Too much jargon has been used.

☐ The hairdresser speaks in a monotone.

All of these can result in:

■ negative impressions;
■ loss of reputation;
■ fewer referrals;
■ static clientele or eventual loss of clients.

## Advantages of improving client consultation skills

☐ You are working to meet clients' needs.

☐ You will enhance your overall practical skills.

☐ Clients will be rewarded.

☐ Job satisfaction will increase.

☐ You will experience less stress when dealing with clients.

- It will encourage the development of greater trust and confidence.

- You will receive more compliments.

- There will be fewer complaints.

- You will win more clients.

## Consultation structure

In order to give your consultations more structure, let us apply the basic selling model, AIDA. Theoretically this represents what you want to achieve during your consultations. In order to reach your objective let us expand the steps, breaking each into a key activity as follows:

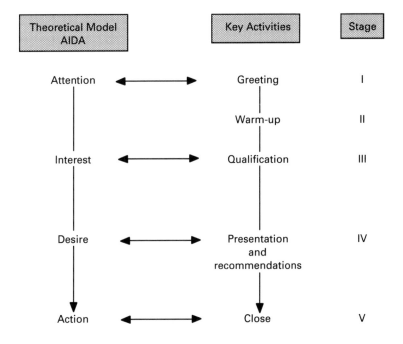

By structuring your consultation in this way, ensuring that you manage each step carefully, fulfilling your objectives, your consultations will take on a professional slickness that is guaranteed to impress clients and bring you referrals.

# Stage I: greeting

Making a positive first impression is vital so take extra care at the initial moment of greeting.

☐ Approach the client in a confident manner, greeting them with a warm friendly smile. Use their name.

☐ Use positive body language such as a firm handshake, eye-to-eye contact and other positive facial expressions. Throughout think about the impression you are making.

☐ Introduce yourself: 'How do you do, my name is . . .', or 'I am very pleased to meet you, my name is . . .'.

☐ If the client is sitting in reception which is away from the main salon area, ask them to follow you: 'Please follow me and take a seat'.

It is sometimes practice to send a trainee to bring a client through into a salon, in which case they should be properly trained to do so. However, I would suggest that, where possible, a stylist should initially greet their own client. If you are running late, go and apologize personally to the client. Make sure they have magazines and coffee. If the client feels they have been forgotten, they will receive a poor impression.

Use these first impressions to assess their emotional state. Watch for body language signals. Assess their overall body style and visual appearance, i.e. your first impressions of them. It will help if the client is *not* wearing a salon gown at this stage. Don't overlook the importance of this stage. Although it may only last seconds, it is vital to both you and your client.

# Stage II: the warm-up

Use this warm-up stage to:

☐ Help your new client adjust to you and the salon atmosphere.

☐ Tell them something about yourself.

☐ Compliment them on a particular aspect of their appearance. Make general smalltalk, e.g. about the weather or who recommended them.

☐ Encourage them to tell you something about themselves.

Further assess their emotional state and personality type. Use your body language skills to complete a more in-depth profile.

## Personality profile

Each client is unique. Consider the following scenario. You are out somewhere special. You look around and observe the people.

- Does any person stand out?
- How would you describe the style of their dress?
- What sort of colours are they wearing?
- How would you describe their hairstyle?
- Are they wearing make-up? If so, how much?
- What is their posture like?
- Can you hear how they are talking?
- Are they using expressive language?

Have you considered how many different personality types are present? Each person is expressing themselves in their own unique way.

Use this technique on your clients, especially new ones, to help you build up a picture in your mind of the type of person you are dealing with. In terms of emotionality would you say they are more extroverted or introverted? This is of course very much a simplification, for, as I discussed earlier (Chapter 6, 'The Real You'), there is always a balance between introversion and extroversion in the well adjusted person.

Try to remain objective even though your impressions may be influenced by your own associations, prejudices and values. Build up a picture of their lifestyle, age, social background, leisure activities, likes and dislikes. This information will be invaluable later. Make notes on their record card.

## Lifestyle considerations

Before you can begin to recommend styles later in the consultation, you will need to consider fully the client's lifestyle on a day-to-day basis, and also appreciate how they may be able to adapt your design for different occasions.

Whether they need a total restyle, a modification to their existing cut, or their hair dressed for a special event, you will need to be aware of the following considerations. Will it be:

- practical?
- manageable?

Lifestyle considerations

| Lifestyle | Considerations | 'Impressions' | Comments |
|---|---|---|---|
| Student | Practical | Adventurous<br>Fashionable | Often the age of experimentation, rebellion and self-expression. Many teenage girls still have long hair which they tend to wear casually. Others may look to role models for inspiration. The young fashion-conscious male is a dedicated follower of current trends. |
| Young married woman with children | Stylish practical cuts<br>Manageable<br>Budget<br>Versatility | Warm<br>Friendly<br>Caring<br>Dependable<br>Fashionable | Time is always an important consideration with the young mother who stays at home to look after the children. She is a woman of many roles. However, there will be occasions when she would like to make a special effort. |
| Young single career woman, e.g. an executive | Practical<br>Manageable<br>Fashionable<br>Versatile<br>Impact<br>Quality | Successful<br>Confident<br>Professional<br>Dynamic<br>Attractive | Appearance is an important issue. Is prepared to spend. Climbing the career ladder plays a major role in her life. Work and socializing tend to follow on from one another, hence the need for a versatile, stylish cut that can be transformed to create different looks. |
| Older woman in business | Softer line<br>Manageable<br>Quality<br>'Well dressed' | Status<br>Sophistication<br>Respectability | The older woman in this instance will most likely rely on a good balance of cutting skills and traditional hairstyling and dressing. Maybe she still visits the hairdressers weekly for a blowdry, set or comb out. |
| Receptionist | Practical<br>Versatile<br>Smart | Friendly<br>Not intimidating<br>Efficient | It is important that as she is on the front line her image is spot on. |
| Single male in a creative career | Practical<br>Stylish cut<br>Fashionable<br>Impact | Creative<br>Ambitious<br>Dynamic<br>Successful<br>Flair | Total look of great importance. Very image conscious. Probably wears short sharp cuts that are cut regularly and groomed using styling products to add to the overall finish. Others may wear their hair longer, possibly tied back. |
| Male in business, commerce or professions | Regular men's cut | Professional<br>Dependable<br>Competent<br>Conservative | Often unadventurous; traditional barbering attitude. |

- appropriate?
- economical to maintain?

Your recommendations should be based on an in-depth lifestyle assessment.

## Good questions to ask:

- Where did they have to travel from?
- How long did it take?
- What type of work do they do?
- What does their work involve?
- Do they have a family?
- Do they have to wear their hair up for work?
- Are there any work restrictions?
- What are their social activities?
- Do they play sport?

## Age considerations

It would certainly be presumptuous to ask a client their age. Judge for yourself. Age is a very important consideration when planning a new hair image. You have probably heard the saying, 'You are as old as you feel'. This is very true. However, most women do not want to look like 'mutton dressed as lamb'. Equally, they do not want to look older than their years unless they have to. A client, male or female, may need to look older for their job, particularly if they have a young face and hold a senior position within a company in charge of a team. They may be perfectly good at their job, but subordinates might resent working under a younger person. Age and style need to be in harmony.

Each time you consult with a client ask yourself:

- Could they look younger?
- Do they need to look older?
- How can you make a client look younger or older?

Build up a record card system for each client. Prepare in advance for each regular client's follow-up appointment using the card as an aid to memory.

Notice how during this stage there is little reference to hair. Use this warm-up stage purely to cement a good relationship with your clients.

Getting it wrong through not using those star qualities, transmitting the wrong signals, creating negative impressions, using poor communication skills, failing to ask questions in a tactful way and failing to listen properly, are all recipes for disaster.

You are more likely to win a client over if they take an immediate liking to you.

# Stage III: qualification

To develop your clients' interest you will need to understand and identify each client's specific needs. In effect the qualification stage is about gathering information, based on a personal and technical evaluation of clients' emotions and needs.

Don't make the mistake of picking up a client's hair between your fingers and exclaiming, with a look of disgust, 'Who cut your hair last time?' The client may reply 'You did!'

Use the qualification stage to state your objectives, and outline your work experience and credentials. Don't forget you are on stage. You will be assessed on your performance.

Tactfully and gently ask relevant questions:

- Find out their objectives.

- Do they have any negative feelings? If so, these need to be tackled later.

- What do they like about their present hairstyle?

- Are there any particular aspects which they are unhappy with?

- Do they have a visual image of how they would like to look? Get them to describe it.

- When did they last have their hair cut?

- Are they happy with the cut?

- Do they want to keep their hair long? If so, how long?

- Do they want to be able to dress their hair occasionally?

- Are they good at styling their hair?

- How much time do they have to do their hair daily?

- If they are in business, would a classic cut be more versatile?

- Are they after a cut that is easy to care for?

- Do they entertain a lot?

☐     Are they going on holiday? If so, where?

☐     Are they planning a special occasion? If so, find out as much as possible about the event, for example:

- The nature of the occasion.
- Time of day.
- Time of year.
- Will it be formal or informal?
- What are they planning to wear?
- If they have long hair, will it be better up or down?

☐     Do they have any important work commitments or engagements such as a job interview, a presentation or a conference?

## Personal evaluation to discover their values, desires and personality profile

By now you will have a clearer idea of:

- What sort of person they are.
- Are they a logical or emotional person?
- Do they need to make a statement?
- Are they looking to you for a new hair direction?
- Is there a need for them to project a powerful image? Will it be appropriate?
- What is their self-esteem like?
- Will they have the confidence to carry a certain look?
- Do they have a fixed idea?
- Will they leave it up to you? (This could be dangerous!)

## Technical evaluation – a visual assessment

How would you describe their hair type, texture, colour, condition and other physical characteristics?

The basis for changing and improving a client's hair image should take into account these physical characteristics, how they interrelate and what affects them. Just as with any material, to get the best out of it it is crucial that you understand how it will perform during all stages of design work. Your style recommendation must be based on:

- an examination of their hairlines and crown for irregular growth patterns;

- how their hair type will react or change during cutting;
- which cutting technique will be the best for their hair texture;
- how, by using the correct hair-care products, the condition of their hair can be improved;
- how colour can visually alter and improve their hair image;
- what permanent waving technique will be most suitable;
- having to grow their hair because at present it is too short.

With a regular client, check their record card in advance for previous service. With a new client, you need to build up a complete profile or case history about their hair and any influencing factors in order to enable you to give them the best professional advice and service. A case history is best built up by asking pertinent questions in line with your observations, such as:

- Do they wear glasses all the time?
- Is their hair coloured?
- If coloured, what was the product used?
- How long ago was their hair coloured?
- Is their hair permed?
- If so, how long ago?
- Have they been in the sun recently?
- Do they swim regularly in a chlorinated pool?
- How often do they wash their hair?
- Do they like to dry their hair naturally?
- Do they use a blow dryer?
- What styling products do they use?
- Does their hair hold a blow dry or set well?
- What styling equipment do they use?
- How long it is since they had a cut?

If you have reason to think that their hair has suffered as a result of their general health or lifestyle, ask such questions as:

- Are they losing much hair?
- Have they been ill recently?
- Are they on any particular medication?
- What is their diet like?
- Do they have much stress in their life?

All these points need to be properly considered and discussed with your clients. It is assumed here that you have a sound technical knowledge.

## Technical evaluation – hair diagnosis

The hair diagnosis is an important aspect of a consultation, reinforcing your hair assessment.

▨ Ask open-ended relevant questions (see section on conversational strategy earlier in this Chapter).

▨ Listen properly to the client's answers.

▨ Physically examine their hair and scalp.

▨ Carry out any tests that you feel are appropriate to find the causes of common problems such as:

- poor elasticity
- over-elasticity
- split ends
- breakage
- rough cuticle
- tangled hair
- dullness
- dryness
- flaky scalp
- faded colour
- poor overall shape.

▨ Continue asking appropriate questions. Think carefully what you plan to say next. Develop a strategy. Learn how to ask the right questions and use the correct words in an agreeable manner. Listen carefully to how the client answers. With experience you will be able to interpret what the client really means.

## Aesthetic evaluation – suitability

Visually assess the relationship between their head, face and body for balance.

▨ Assess their face shape, facial features, profile, neck length, width and shoulder dimensions.

- Consider proportion, line and balance and discuss how, by working with these aesthetic considerations, you can enhance their facial features.

▨ If you are proposing to recommend a colouring service, have you taken into consideration the client's unique colour profile:

- The depth of the client's natural hair colour, i.e. how light or dark are they?
- What are the undertones in their hair? Are they warm or cool?
- How light or dark is their skin? What is its colour value?
- How warm or cool is their skin tone?
- Do they have much contrast between their hair and skin tones? This clarity will determine how bright or soft their hair colour needs to be.

Undertone, intensity and clarity are terms that an artist uses to describe colour. When applied to the tonal system of colour analysis they give us a very good diagnostic tool to assess a client's colour profile and extend our understanding of colour aesthetics. (For those of you who would like to know more about this system and advance your colouring services, please refer to Appendix 2 on Ian Mistlin's consultancy services.)

If this qualification stage is rushed or you fail to ask the right questions, you may risk making wrong assumptions. Once you are satisfied that you have gathered sufficient information, you will be in a good position to present your recommendations, tailor your services to the client individually and bring the consultation to a close.

Customizing the consultation to each client's wants and needs will show you really care. Once your client realizes this, their interest will grow and they are more likely to be receptive to your ideas and perceive that you are offering a service that is of true value to them.

# Stage IV: presentation and recommendations

The purpose of the presentation in the consultation is to give the client sufficient feedback from the information you have gathered to help them make a style decision or buy other salon services/products that will be of benefit and advantage to them, then moving them to the desire stage of the AIDA model.

Throughout the qualification stage I'm sure your client will have been keen to ask questions. Use Stage IV to give the client an opportunity to express their opinions and feelings. Naturally you must respond.

Learn to anticipate the type of questions clients ask, or would like to ask and yet may never do so. Use this technique to impress your clients:

HAIRDRESSER:   I'm sure you will like to know how you can improve your hair condition . . .

Your aim should be to draw each client into this stage, so they feel that they are involved in the decision process.

Your presentation should be tailored to each client's personality, values, needs and desires.

- Are they extroverted or introverted?
- What is their self-image?
- Do they lack confidence? If so, confidence build.
- Listen with empathy.
- Use all your star qualities to move their emotional state into feeling good about themselves.

Help them to visualize how good they will look. Many clients find it difficult to imagine how a style will look when finished. Some may bring a photograph with them. This may not be the best style for them; however, don't be abrupt or aggressive about it. Use it as a starting point to introduce your presentation. If it helps, build up a portfolio of styles that you can use to make the presentation as visual as possible.

Give the client a number of style options. State why the looks you have recommended will be better for them. Give reasons.

Emphasize services of special interest and value. If you consider that a hair treatment will help to improve their overall hair condition, advise them accordingly and support your claim with facts.

Increase your clients' hair awareness through education. Discuss how to look after their hair, and what products will be compatible for their hair type and texture.

Discuss features and benefits of your recommendations. Qualify a feature with the words 'What this means to you is . . .'.

If the client shows interest by asking about a service, be enthusiastic. For example, if the client asks about colour, discuss what technique would be most suitable to enhance the cut or liven up their hair. Use expressive words to heighten their good feelings.

Be honest if you consider a client's request is unsuitable for whatever reason. Back this up with your reasons and then come up with a positive alternative.

Balance the technical aspects of your presentation with a creative element. This way you are sure to appeal to those clients who make decisions based on logic compared with those clients who respond to emotional values.

☐ Employ active listening techniques combined with paraphrasing to confirm a client's understanding and liking for your recommendations. Use this at a suitable point in the presentation to bring it to a climax, by getting the client to agree.

☐ Do not forget, be embarrassed or be frightened about discussing money. The client needs to know in advance what your services or products will cost them. They may have a tight budget, or not have sufficient funds or even credit cards with them.

☐ Make your presentations fun and exciting. Reward each client with positive, expressive, facial and body language as you consider appropriate. Vary your vocal tone to heighten your enthusiasm and decisiveness, moving the client towards the final stage of the consultation, the close.

## Visualization

It is important during the presentation stage that you are able to convey your ideas and paint a clear picture using precise, non-technical language so that the client is fully aware, before any service commences, of what you mean and appreciates your advice.

Make sure, for instance, that you understand what the client means by such phrases as:

'I only want a trim.'
'I would like a short cut.'
'Not too short.'
'A curly perm.'

These phrases are riddled with danger signals, signalling the need to be more exact.

Explain the proposed new style as a benefit to them. For example, it will:

- make them look years younger;
- enhance their bone structure;
- show off their eyes;
- make their hair easier to handle;
- improve their hair colour;
- make them look more sexy.

Lastly, have you built up a picture in your mind of how the finished cut/

style will look? Has the client a firm idea of what the end result will look like? Are you confident you can do it? Is the client confident?

## Summary

Here are the important points to remember:

- Learn to ask the right questions.

- Be sure that you are listening correctly in order that you understand fully what type of style they are after.

- If they want to keep the length, how much and why?

- Do they want an easy to care for style?

- Watch their body language.

- Be aware of your own body language.

- Do not be dismissive of their ideas.

- Do not make them feel guilty about their hair.

- Do not be aggressive or get frustrated.

- Do not let clients think you are doing them a favour.

- Listen to constructive comments.

- Accept valid objections.

- Make sure you consider all of a client's needs.

- Make sure you are both speaking the same language.

- Have confidence in your judgement. Stick to your decision: if you consider that a client's style wishes are unsuitable, say so tactfully. Give them a positive alternative.

# Stage V: the close (decision time)

This is the climax to the consultation, when the client gives definite buying signals. If you close too soon, you will be seen as too pushy. You should close only when you are sure you can help the client satisfy their needs and can produce the results. Trust is essential and has to be firmly established. A client will have more respect for you if you are honest and say, 'I cannot meet your needs', rather than build up their expectations unfairly.

## What are the buying signals?

There are both verbal and non-verbal buying signals. The more experienced you become in using communication skills, the easier it will be to recognize the signals.

### Verbal signals

- The client answers your questions positively.
- They agree with what you say.
- The client shows interest and asks questions.
- They talk positively about using a product.

> 'When I use the . . . do I . . .?'
> 'How much should I use?'
> 'How often will I need my hair cut to keep it in shape?'
> 'After I have had my hair cut, what type of highlights would you recommend?'

- Client asks such questions as:

> 'Can I pay using a credit card?'
> 'How long will it take to do?'

Time may become an objection. If necessary, suggest that the client make another appointment for a particular service. Go with them to the reception in order to ensure that the right amount of time is allocated and that the correct booking procedure is followed.

If appropriate, arrange for tests to be carried out before the main appointment. This means better time management for everyone concerned.

### Non-verbal signals

- The client sits more forward in the chair in anticipation.
- Eye contact. Their pupils will be slightly more dilated, which indicates interest.
- Positive facial expressions, such as smiling, using the head cocked to show they are listening.
- A relaxed brow.

- The arms are uncrossed, with the palms of the hands placed gently on their lap.
- The legs are uncrossed.
- The client sits forwards resting the chin on the hand.
- They show interest by picking up a product.
- They look at themselves in the mirror with interest.

When you feel you have the orange light, this is the best time to ask. Then wait for the green light.

- 'As you are happy with my recommendations, can I get an assistant to shampoo your hair?'
- 'I'm very pleased to see you are excited at my ideas. Can I take you through into the . . . department for . . .?'
- 'Would you like to purchase the products I have recommended? I know you will be thrilled at how good they are.'
- 'Would you like to make a booking for a follow-up appointment in four weeks?'
- 'Would you like to restyle your hair now?'
- 'Can I proceed?'

*If you don't ask, you might never know.*

# Dealing with a client's objections

Situations in which you have to deal with a client's doubts, objections and obstacles to your recommendations should be expected and welcomed. I would be concerned during a consultation if objections never arose. An apathetic client would worry me. This could be a sure sign that:

- You have failed to impress.
- You have failed to attract, excite and stimulate their interest sufficiently.

It may mean that they cannot understand or visualize what you have recommended. If, after your presentation, the client says, 'Well, I'll leave it up to you,' proceed with caution. This may imply that:

- They have full trust and confidence in your judgement.
- They are indecisive.
- They do not want to be responsible for the decision.

They may come up with another statement or excuse that implies that they are unsure of the true value of your services or products to them. The trick is not to get frustrated but gently overcome their objections by:

- Applying an active listening and paraphrasing technique.
- Asking appropriate questions to ensure you fully understand.
- Appearing to accept their point of view. This will convince the client that you understand their feelings. 'I understand how you feel . . .'.
- Smiling.
- Adjusting the tone of voice to match theirs.
- Matching their mood.
- Using the head nod and head cock when listening.
- Don't get defensive, angry or flustered. Stay patient.

The closer you can get to knowing your client's real feelings and fears, the easier it will be to neutralize them in exchange for features and benefits of true value.

Building value through empathy will encourage your clients to perceive that what you are offering far outweighs their reasons for not immediately buying your recommendations.

## Reasons for objections

It would be unnatural if you did not expect clients to have valid objections. When out shopping for, say, a new outfit, do you buy the first item that is offered to you? I'm sure you don't. Likewise clients will have genuine worries about:

- Whether they are ready for a dramatic change.
- What happens if they don't like the finished result.
- Whether the cut might be too short and not suit them, or whether a perm might be too curly.
- What family and friends might say.
- Restrictions imposed by their partner.
- The fact that the hair might take a long time to grow again.
- The fear of change after many years.

In these instances you will need to be extra sensitive to their lack of self-confidence. Probe gently. Practise confidence building to reduce their fears, starting by making them feel good about themselves.

Some clients may not be totally convinced at first. They might need further reassurance before they fully trust you.

> CLIENT: It sounds like the cut will be too short.
>
> HAIRDRESSER: It will be shorter, to just above your shoulders, the length and bluntness of the cut will make your hair much thicker, sharper and more flattering for your bone structure.

**Useful words.** 'Yes, but' are useful words to use to turn an objection around by outlining positive benefits.

> HAIRDRESSER: Why do you think it will be too short?

Asking 'why' gets the client to answer their own objections.

> CLIENT: I need to be able to tie my hair back for sport.

**Give them testimonials.** Use previous clients' testimonials to draw reference to how they felt about your services.

> HAIRDRESSER: Can you see that client sitting over there? She had the same concern as you last week. I cut her hair to the same length as I am suggesting for you. She's thrilled with it and has had lots of compliments. She has come back to have some highlights.

Some clients may think they do not have a need for a particular service or product. For example:

> CLIENT: I already use a shampoo and conditioner I bought from ...

Your reply should be based on finding out what products they are using and on pointing out the value of your specialized hair-care range, its unique selling features, and the benefits to the client. Draw comparisons but don't knock. To do this effectively you will need to be familiar with other brand names.

**Sensing the goods.** Let the client see the product and even smell it. At the backwash let them touch their hair and feel how good it feels.
   If the client is still unsure and you have sample sachets, give them some to find out for themselves. What better way to win a client over than to let them experience the benefits first hand?

**Building value.** When it comes to building up the value of your services or products, tell clients how they are going to benefit from what you are recommending. Mention a feature and introduce benefits using the words, 'What this means to you is ...'. For example:

> HAIRDRESSER: The colour I recommend you to use is a semi-permanent. What this means to you is that besides adding richness to

your natural hair colour, you will not have to worry about a regrowth every month.

If, after listening to a client's objections, you get the impression that they have not fully understood, recap on your presentation. Subtly probe to find out how the breakdown in communication occurred.

- **Buying smokescreens.** A client may often raise objections which you consider to be invalid and only a smokescreen for the real reason, which is as yet unclear. You may never discover it. Perhaps they cannot afford the service and are embarrassed to say so. With experience you will be able to read between the lines. Be sensitive to these issues.

- **The 'Yes-but' client.** Beware of the 'Yes, but...' client who continually raises objections. If you consider you have reached a stalemate situation or have a difficult client that you cannot handle, don't get annoyed. Stay calm. Support your case logically and emotionally. If necessary, get advice from the manager, artistic director or head technician.

- **A client's prerogative.** Remember: it is the client's prerogative to say no or 'I want to think it over'. You must not bully them into making a decision that they may regret. A cool-off period may be the best answer for both of you.

## The price factor

One of the most common objections raised by a client about buying services or products is about price. Don't avoid the issue of money. At some stage in your presentation a client will need to know about cost. In a competitive economic market clients will be basing their spending on perceived quality and value for money. Base your selling on value, not price. Stress the benefits to them.

Approach the issue confidently. If you believe that what you are offering is of true value, if you believe that the products you recommend will be of true benefit, then the client will be more convinced. If you seem nervous or try to evade this issue, it may alarm your client into questioning your honesty.

When a client comments on or objects to prices, they may mean that:

- They genuinely do not have the money.
- They have not budgeted to pay as much.
- They have an unrealistic idea of the true value of your service.

- You have not succeeded in convincing them.
- They have not fully appreciated the real benefits.
- They are comparing you with a competitor and they perceive the value of your services as less attractive.
- They are confused by your pricing policy and scale of charges.
- They are trying to haggle over your fees in order to get a bargain.
- They are using price as a smokescreen for some other objection.

## Overcoming price objections

Use the objection as a way to explore reasons:

> CLIENT: I was not expecting to pay so much for my highlights.
> HAIRDRESSER: Do you mind if I ask you how much you were expecting to spend?
> CLIENT: I know I can get my highlights done for . . .
> HAIRDRESSER: Tell me, is that for half a head or a whole head? Are they foil highlights or cap highlights? How many colours would they use?

Anticipate questions, and then give answers to justify the reasons for the variations and to support your case. Use a feature and its benefits to politely say that 'one only gets for what one pays for'.

> HAIRDRESSER: I hope this has helped you to make up your mind. Would you like me/us to do the highlights for you?

Introduce an additional benefit and then close the sale.

## Consultation and buying summary

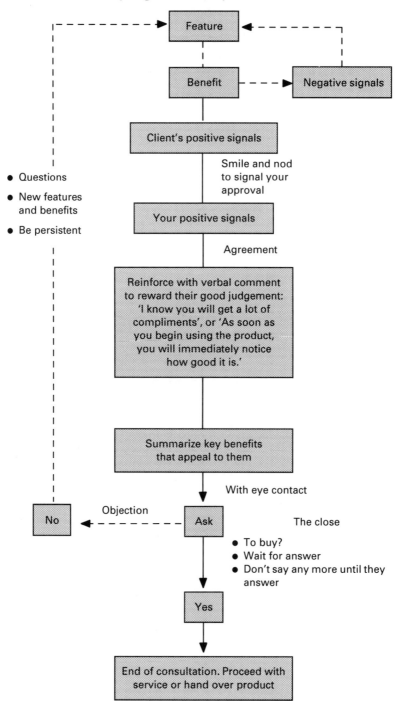

# PART V
# NURTURING A QUALITY CULTURE

# 10
# A Route for Change

## Introduction

Hairdressing is an adventure, a lifetime journey that is rich in rewards. However, unless care is taken, there are many pitfalls en route. It is said that history contains the key to the future. However, it is all very well reflecting on the past. It is easy to be wise after the event and with hindsight to realize the mistakes made. We can all make excuses as to how things should have been. However, can we plan a preventative business strategy for the future so as to ensure that history does not repeat itself?

As we look forwards, what will the future have in store for you? What will be the future for the industry, and what changes will need to be made?

Change is what governments worldwide are looking for as they tackle a wide range of economic and social issues. Sustained progress will only be made by developing a society with a culture based on *quality* in every activity from health care to business. It will only be achieved by educating people to understand the benefits to them personally and to society as a whole, and must be supported by a programme of continuous training.

Many organizations and businesses are also looking at adopting a quality culture as the way forward. So what about hairdressing?

The following are my essential recommendations for changes, based on my observations and evaluations. You may not agree with them immediately, but don't dismiss them lightly. Think them through. Use them to open up constructive discussions between team members. Access your own resources and brainstorm your ideas in order to develop your business objectives. Formulate an action plan of priorities. However, be patient. Don't rush into making sweeping changes without first communicating them to the team. Go about it in a controlled way and remember that a change for the better need not necessarily be dramatic; even the smallest change can often make a substantial improvement.

# Looking forward

## *Perfect your marketing*

Fulfil your business objectives by developing a clear marketing plan based on a client-centred approach to marketing. Your strategy should be drawn up with military precision, and must focus on identifying market opportunities, clients' needs, your resources and the best way to communicate your message. Your plan should be reviewed and revised regularly with a view to continuous improvement.

## *Educate your clients*

When it comes to communicating your message, don't overlook the importance of personal selling. Too little importance is attached to the consultation and accompanying skills in hairdressing today. Is this because of the time factor? Is this because traditionally it is given free? You can go to your local doctor's surgery when you are ill, wait and eventually be seen by a doctor who has little time to spend talking to you, or you can pay and go privately and get a longer consultation time. The solution is to change your consultation system.

## *Encourage team pride*

Encourage individual team players and the team as a unit to take pride in their skills and services by giving them the framework that enables them to do so. The framework should be built around recognizing the importance in a quality culture of the team as a well oiled structure that is actively involved in managing the needs of clients.

Each team player and service interface must be encouraged to see themselves as 'management satellites' within the team infrastructure. This requires them to assume a responsibility for quality management. In this way each team member has a role to play in planning, running and standard setting within the salon over and above their other duties. This will contribute significantly towards ensuring individual job satisfaction and improving team performance.

## *Preach individual quality control*

Build a system that incorporates quality control naturally into the manufacture stage of each hair design. It will be far more profitable to teach team players the benefits of good workmanship and to monitor their own results before the client leaves the salon.

## Give positive feedback and praise

Every team player needs feedback in order to know how well they are doing. So does the team as a whole. A pat on the back costs nothing yet it is a powerful motivator in setting standards and encouraging good performance. It says that you noticed. To help team players to reach their full potential, catch them doing something right rather than remarking only on things they do wrong.

## Encourage ambition

Every person needs goals. The team needs to focus on achieving results. Help them to fulfil their goals by realistic goal setting.

## Nurture perfection

Instil into your team the need to strive for perfection. Encourage each team player to continuously improve their skills and services. Hold regular practice sessions to encourage the cross-fertilization of new ideas and provide an opportunity for everyone to perfect their technique.

## Remove team blind spots

It is essential that everyone within the team appreciates one another's responsibilities and problems in order to ensure that barriers are not formed. Such barriers would only lead to the destabilization of the team structure and team performance. Teams should be built with balance in mind: the right balance of different personalities.

## Develop the potential of people managing

We must move away from the manager who needs to be in control, who interprets the position as 'managing people' and exerting authority.

We need to evolve a culture of creative salon management in which the manager or owner becomes a facilitator and negotiator skilled in the 'potential of people managing'.

The difference may appear very subtle. However, there is a very big difference between managing people and people managing. Quality management is built around developing a resourceful team that can manage itself. Here we have a leader rather than a manager. The leader operates from the very heart of the team on the shop floor, focusing, energizing, identifying new directions, planning how to bring about change for the better and taking positive action. In this new role the leader is a conductor and the team the orchestra. To lead you will not need a baton, but you will need expert communication skills.

## Remove complacency

The aim is to turn client behaviour into positive consequences. Strive to keep your clients coming back for a considerable length of time. Whether or not they do so will depend on how well you reward them.

It will not stop there. The client merry-go-round will continue to turn in your favour through referrals. Through each rewarded client, others will get to hear of your excellent services and follow. Just watch your clientele grow. News of your reputation will travel fast, customers will flock to use your services and client volume will grow rapidly. Soon you will have more business than you can handle. Clients may have to wait. Perhaps next time the service will not be quite so good.

The truth is you are only as good as that moment in time. It will not be long before the quality of service and skills will be affected. Complacency may set in. The bubble may be about to burst. You may not see it coming. You may blame everyone and everything, but unless you get to grips with the real reasons and face up to the truth, even though it might be painful, your business or how you work may be locked in a stranglehold, doomed to die a slow death.

## Design a fair reward system

Throughout the book I have been talking about rewarding the client. What about rewarding team players or the team as a whole for a job well done? Undoubtedly at some time the question will be asked, 'What is in it for me?'. That's a fair question, and one that needs a fair answer if you are looking to achieve better and better results. We have talked about features, benefits and desire.

- What are the features in the team members' jobs?
- What are the benefits to them?
- What will give them the desire to continually perform well?

There is a simple equation:

Rewarded staff = Rewarded clients

If you do not reward your staff, the balance of the equation will be upset.

If we are to reward staff for keeping and winning clients, i.e. for client satisfaction, we need to consider a reward and incentive system that:

- is fair to everyone (the business, each player and the team);
- is easy to understand;
- ensures that individuals can influence the desired outcome;
- produces results that are measurable;
- means that the rewards are easy to pay and can be paid at regular intervals.

We are all aware of the traditional wage structures that operate within salons, based on productivity and the time worked. They can include:

- a basic wage structure;
- a straight commission scheme;
- commission on retail sales;
- commission on technical sales.

It is outside the scope of the book to discuss the mechanics of these or the merits for and against particular wage structures and whether these operate separately or as a joint package. There are two important questions that need to be asked, however, namely:

- Do they measure quality?
- Do they consider team performance?

We need to consider reward systems that are linked to client satisfaction targets and that are paid to the team and to individual team players. For such a system to be fair, options must be discussed and agreed with the team.

## Increase responsibilities

If individuals do not feel that they are progressing within a salon or company, either through promotion or through being given increased responsibilities, they are likely to get restless.

## Promote further education

This is a great tool for increasing job motivation. It gives individuals opportunities to further their knowledge and acquire new skills.

## Offer a piece of the action

This is the ultimate reward that may encourage a key member to stay, so consider offering a partnership or profit-sharing scheme.

## Remove that tunnel vision

Imagine looking at life through a narrow tunnel. Your vision will be greatly restricted, although you may be still able to see something at the other end. Now remove the tunnel. Your field of view will now be much greater. You will be able to see more activity taking place around you.

Apply this to making sure that you know what is happening in the world outside your salon. When it comes to dealing with people and problems, keep an open mind; look, listen and evaluate before you respond. Be flexible and creative in your decision making and when developing your own style.

## Institute training

Throughout the book I have consistently talked about clients' needs, but what about the needs of individual team members? Are they confident they can deliver the goods or service? Is the client, and, most of all, are you? Consider how you would answer these questions.

- Do you engage casual staff to help on busy days?
- Do you get a newly recruited apprentice to shampoo a client without first showing them the procedure?
- Do you employ and put to work hairdressers without first evaluating their skills?
- Do you have stylists who make excuses or shy away from performing certain services simply because they are unsure about how to carry them out or cannot do so?
- Do you have unqualified stylists carrying out cutting on paying clients?
- Do you have a staff member who is struggling in a position of responsibility?
- Do you have a trainee to answer the telephone who is unskilled in reception procedure?

The list could go on and on. Consider, too, how many unhappy clients you may lose each week, month or year simply because you:

- take it for granted that a person is fit and able to do the job;
- allow a person to start work without an induction programme of basic skills training;
- fail to recognize the need to continuously update standards of work.

If you want your staff to perform as a team, you need to give them the 'basic equipment' to tackle and solve problems that will arise daily on the shop floor. You need to train and educate them so they are able to make their own decisions and are confident about doing so.

You must aim to unlock and utilize the full potential in every member as part of a continuous improvement strategy through:

**Skills training.** Giving each person the complete 'tools' and more to do the job.

**Shop-floor training.** Where better place to instruct than in the working environment?

**Soirées or practice sessions.** An excellent environment for encouraging the cross-fertilization of ideas, and a chance to practise new techniques.

**Retraining.** A policy of revitalization, giving staff the chance to assess and update their standards of hairdressing and their management skills.

## Develop a system that values time

Improving quality means improving the production system. We need to look at how the goods are delivered to the client from the moment they enter the salon to the time they leave. We need to look at how we can utilize time more effectively. This does not mean we must get faster and faster at the expense of quality. What it means is that we must look at how efficiently time is managed if the service to clients is to be continuously improved.

If you leave a tap running at the backwash, by the end of the day just imagine how much water would have been wasted. The simple solution would be to turn off the tap.

Time, unlike the tap, cannot be shut off: the minutes tick by and turn into hours, and so on. Think of the amount of time wasted. We value time and feel good when we use it productively, but become frustrated and annoyed if it is used unproductively. I'm sure you have been in situations in which you have had to wait for a train, queued up in the supermarket, waited in a traffic jam, or even spent hours looking for something. I know how annoyed you must have felt. Now you can appreciate how a client feels when they have to wait and waste their time.

Clients' time is wasted if:

- They are kept waiting at reception to book in.
- They are kept waiting because a mistake has been made in the booking.
- The stylist is still with the previous client and will be for some time.
- There is a bottleneck of clients due to overbooking.
- They have to wait for a shampoo to be done because there are no trainees.
- Staff have to search for clean towels.
- They have to wait for a vacant chair.
- They have to wait because there are insufficient hair dryers.
- They have to wait for a stylist to supervise after a trainee has blowdried a client.
- They have to wait because the sequence of different stages in the client's service has been booked incorrectly.
- They have to wait for a cup of coffee which in the end arrives late and cold.
- They are made to wait to pay at reception because the bill is nowhere to be found or has not been filled in properly.

Again, the list could go on. It highlights the everyday problems that can and do occur.

Planning your services to eliminate time wasting will give you a tremendous competitive advantage. It may be difficult to redesign your system, but it will cost you nothing except your time and the rewards will soon be apparent. Your clients will respond well and so will your team.

Work with your team at:

- Improving your booking and administration procedures.
- Streamlining routine jobs.
- Maintaining effective communication.
- Ensuring that materials are in the right place and that stock is kept above a certain level.
- Ensuring that equipment is well maintained.
- Making certain that the team mechanics are well oiled.
- Ensuring that team members are flexible and are willing to help one another.

■ Evaluating the layout of the salon so that sites for locating services such as backwashes, refreshment areas, dispensary, laundry, cloakroom and reception are situated within easy reach. Delays can occur if staff have to work in a badly designed salon.

■ Making sure that the salon is orderly and that everyone recognizes that tidiness is a product of a quality system.

## Evaluate your appointment system

■ Is the frequency of your appointments designed to encourage overproduction, bottlenecks, bad timing and client waiting?

■ Are you booking beyond a capacity at which you can cope?

■ Is overbooking causing bottlenecks within the system?

■ Have you investigated at which stage in the client's service the bottleneck is occurring?

■ Once you have established the source of bottlenecks, what can you do about it so as not to disrupt and damage the service?

■ Have you considered that each service needs to be allocated sufficient time to complete it to a quality standard? For example, a restyle on a new client is going to take longer than a four- to six-weekly cut on a regular client; and a blowdry on long thick hair is certainly going to take longer than a short-hair blowdry. Do you plan for such contingencies?

Extending the length of appointment times for different services would certainly be advantageous to everyone. However, there must be consultation between the client, the reception and the stylist. The client needs to be asked over the phone when booking what services they require, the type of hair, its length and so on, by a receptionist who understands the importance of this job and who is capable of estimating the amount of time that will be needed. This approach will help to reduce delays caused by unpredictable events that might arise on the day.

## Improve consistency

This may well be the factor that determines whether a client decides to stay with you or go elsewhere. Don't let your competition get an advantage by allowing your standard of work or service to fluctuate each time clients visit you. Keep your standards consistently high.

## Charge realistic fees

If we are to elevate overall standards within the industry, clients must be educated to appreciate quality. They must recognize that long-term investment is necessary if we are to

- improve the quality of work and of service;
- tailor the length of appointments to suit their particular needs;
- spend more time on them personally if the need should arise.

However, all investments need to be funded initially. We must be willing to fund them with our time and resources, but clients must be willing to pay realistically for this quality. They must respect a non-fixed scale of fees geared towards delivering a personal service rather than manufacturing a standard product.

## We must believe that all staff are productive

If we are to nurture client-focused teams, we must develop the philosophy that all staff are productive and have a vital contribution to make in a quality culture.

## Man the front line

Don't ignore the critical role that the reception area plays in a service-driven industry. It is the first and last interface to deal with managing the client's needs. If you are operating without a receptionist or with inadequately trained reception staff, then you may cut your overheads in the short term but will greatly reduce your profits in the long term.

## Set realistic targets

If we are to develop a quality culture, we must improve standards. I am not talking about average standards but high ones. 'Average' must cease to be a term we use. However, many target measurements are based on worker averages, for example average clients per day or per month. True, these calculations do measure how many clients an operator can deal with in a fixed period of time. However, a number of factors can determine worker productivity, for example:

- how many clients the worker is 'fed';
- how fast they work;

- the nature of the service;
- each client's needs;
- how much time and care the operator invests;
- how much each person is charged, i.e. your fees;
- the level of support the worker gets from the system.

It is all very well saying to an operator, 'You will need to increase your client volume by $x$%', but do you discuss how they will do so? We must look at our systems to ensure that they are fair to each operator and are not simply sacrificing quality for short-term productivity.

## The need for change

Whether salons in the future will be successful and profitable or unsuccessful will hinge on their standards of excellence in fulfilling the needs of their clients.

How can we use our time, our talents and those of our staff, and other resources more effectively to ensure that we build a stronger, more resilient business that will be resistant to market forces and that will enable us to improve sales yield and increase our profits?

The answer lies in the roots that support your business structure. Like the roots of a giant oak tree, strength will depend on personal development, how well teams are motivated and how far you are prepared to go in building a quality structure that has the client at the centre.

Are you confident in succeeding? Is there anything holding you back?

- Are you limiting your success through negative beliefs?
- Are you frightened of change?
- Do you fear failure?
- Do you shy away from problems?
- Do you encourage team performance?

If you are to bring about change you must move towards developing a positive self and positive teams not hampered by limiting beliefs. Do not be scared of success: you must be physically and mentally equipped to take on new challenges with relish, thinking both logically and intuitively in developing true potential.

# *Appendix 1*
# *NVQs*

*How to Win Clients and Interpret their Needs* is about raising standards. My concern for high standards means that I am very heartened by the introduction of the National Vocational Qualifications or NVQs, the aim of which is to train more people to higher levels so that they can produce quality products and services.

The NVQ scheme is based on a framework of five levels of achievement with Level 1 being the simplest. Each level is made up of units of competence; each unit is made up of a number of elements describing required performance criteria.

If you are working on the following elements to obtain qualifications in levels 2, 3 and 4, you will find *How to Win Clients and Interpret their Needs* essential and stimulating reading. For easy reference I have included the following table giving details of the units and elements which are covered by the book.

To those of you who are keen to obtain these qualifications in hairdressing, good luck! I know in time your personal investment will be rewarded.

| Level | Unit | Unit description | Element | Element description |
|---|---|---|---|---|
| 2 | 02 | Consulting clients and diagnosing hair and scalp conditions. | 02.01 to 02.12 | Refer to HTB handbook for complete breakdown of respective performance criteria. |
| | 11 | Selling salon services | 11.02 | Comparing and describing the benefits of a defined range of products and commodities. |
| | | | 11.03 | Identifying clients' characteristics and targeting products/services appropriately. |
| | | | 11.04 | Taking advantage of opportunities presented by the presence of clients in a salon to offer additional services and commodities. |

| Level | Unit | Unit description | Element | Element description |
|---|---|---|---|---|
| 3 | B.2 | Establish and maintain effective relationships with clients. | B.2.1 | Promote and develop effective relationships with clients. |
| | | | B.2.2 | Investigate and deal with client complaints within one's area of responsibility. |
| | C.1 | Monitor and maintain client consultation systems and procedures. | C.1.1 | Consult with and advise clients on technical services products and after care. |
| 4 | A.1 | Establish and control systems and procedures to support the provision of a quality service. | A.1.2 | Establish and control client consultation systems and procedures. |
| | | | A.1.3 | Establish, maintain and improve the business image. |
| | | | A.4.1 | Maintain client service according to market position and/or pre-determined standards. |
| | | | B.1.1 | Establish market position as a basis for the development of a business plan. |
| | | | B.1.3 | Review and evaluate agreed business plans and strategies against actual performance. |

Please refer to the respective Hairdressing Training Board booklets for more detailed information about performance criteria and range statements.

# Appendix 2
# Ian Mistlin's Consultancy Services

For details on Ian Mistlin's hairdressing consultancy services, personal development and skills training programmes please photocopy and complete this form and send to:

IAN MISTLIN
IMAGE MATTERS
TEL: 071-581 8864

Name   : _____

Salon   : _____

Address  : _____

_____

_____ Phone No. _____

Position  : _____

I am interested in (please tick)

Consultancy Services for Salons  ☐

Personal Development Workshops  ☐

Skills Training, Open Programmes  ☐

In-House Programmes  ☐

Individual Consultations  ☐

Colour and Image Training  ☐

# *Index*